THE HEALERS

Triumphs, Tragedies, and Tears

How people of diverse talents and intentions advanced or impeded the art and science of healing

Kenneth Maxwell

Cover design: Rita Toews

Cover image: © OriGene Technologies, Inc. Used with permission.

Formatted by Polgarus Studio

CONTENTS

Acknowledgments i
Introduction iii

Part I Early Healers 1
    1. Gods, Kings, And Doctors 3
    2. Hippocrates 8
    3. Galen 13
    4. Healers Of The Middle Ages 16

Part II The Scientific Revolution 19
    5. Seeing The Unseeable 21
    6. Heart And Blood 25
    7. Pasteur 28
    8. The Explorer 37
    9. The Immunizers 41
    10. Pasteur's Vaccination 45
    11. Of Peas And People 52

Part III Battle Against Insects 57
    12. Insects And Diseases 59
    13. Bad Air 62
    14. Yellow Jack 72
    15. A Lousy War 77
    16. Plagues And The Plague 83

Part IV Drugs 91
    17. Wonder Drugs 93
    18. Mad Microbes 99
    19. Right And Left Of Medicines 104
    20. FDA—The 300 Year War 110
    21. A Chinese Puzzle 117
    22. A Bloody Shame 121

Part V Healthful Living 127
23. Sanitation 129
24. The Solution 136
25. The Water War 140
26. Feeders And Breeders 146

Part VI Humanity 157
27. Madness 159
28. Improving Mankind 169
29. Weeding The Unfit 172
30. The Master Race 177
31. Good From Evil 180
32. The Bargain 184

Part VII Mice 193
33. Of Mice And Medicine 195
34. Human Mice And The Gulf War 199

Part VIII Healing And The Mind 207
35. Fountain Of Youth 209
36. The Power Of Belief 215
37. Faith Healers 220
38. Mesmerism 228
39. Biofeedback 234
40. A Self Healer 239

References 243
About The Author 265

ACKNOWLEDGMENTS

My special thanks to Dr. Greayer Mansfield-Jones and Jennifer Mansfield-Jones for their reviewing an early version of the manuscript and for offering many valuable suggestions.

Lynn McGowan was helpful in many ways besides retyping the entire manuscript in Microsoft Word, a form more suitable for the plan of publishing the document. She was helpful in suggesting improvements in the cover design and obtaining permission for their use. She also offered illustrations for possible use in the body of the book. Thus, she provided both a finished document in print plus hard drive copies for use in editing and possible revisions.

The cover design was by Rita Teows. The cover image was copyrighted by OriGene Technologies, Inc., used with permission.

I am deeply grateful to my daughter, Carolyn, for her careful and thorough editing the manuscript and making suggestions during this work. The book could not have come into existence without her timely and sturdy support at every step of the way. I relied on her advice and support. She also supervised and managed the formatting and printing. I thank you, from the bottom of my heart.

The book contains information derived from numerous sources listed in "references". By far the most dependable source was the great science historian Isaac Asimov in his *Asimov's Biographical Encyclopedia of Science and Technology, Second Revised Edition*, Doubleday & Company, Inc., Garden City, New York. 1982.

INTRODUCTION

The Healers tells how people of different talents and intentions dealt with diseases and health. It tells how many of the greatest contributions to human health were made by people who did not prescribe pills or wield scalpels. Some had medical credentials, many did not. They were chemists, physicists, botanists, microbiologists, entomologists, engineers, psychologists, and people with a variety of other interests.

Epidemics raged for centuries during which both victims and wanna-be healers were mired in imaginative superstitions about causes. Treatments generally were a mixed bag of remedies that were sometimes beneficial but mostly harmful or useless. Some inevitably killed more patients than they cured.

While it's necessary and desirable for explanatory reasons to discuss diseases, their causes, origins, symptoms, and treatments, the primary focus of the book is on people, their backgrounds, personalities, qualifications, and accomplishments. It tells how they got it right. It tells how some went wrong. It tells how others, some with medical credentials, victimized men, women and children to satisfy their self-serving ambitions and social causes. To emphasize the importance of people, good or bad, their names are written in boldface.

The Healers is in eight parts covering forty, mostly short, chapters. For example, topics include the recurring battle against insect vectors of disease, about the FDA's tussle with developers of drugs, which can kill or cure, about ambitious and cruel steps to allegedly improve humanity, about experiments on fellow humans, about the interface of mind and health, and much more.

I selectively present the personalities, qualifications and accomplishments of people who made important contributions, for better or worse, to the health and well-being of humanity. Most of the healers were competent or well-meaning. Some were saintly, some were evil. You, dear reader, can decide.

Kenneth E. Maxwell, Ph.D.

PART I
EARLY HEALERS

1 GODS, KINGS, AND DOCTORS

2 HIPPOCRATES

3 GALEN

4 HEALERS OF THE MIDDLE AGES

CHAPTER 1

GODS, KINGS, AND DOCTORS

The greatest healer of ancient times was **Imhotep**, an Egyptian who ruled the country under the patronage of **King Zoser** who reigned over Egypt in the third dynasty (2700 to 2200 B.C.). Imhotep was remarkably talented in a number of roles. Born to a family of architects, he designed and built the first step-pyramid at the modern village of Sakkara, near the site of ancient Memphis. It was intended as King Zoser's tomb. As viceroy, Imhotep was Chief Priest, Chief Justice, Astronomer and Magician of the king's court. He was thought of as a great sage and scribe.

Imhotep's most notable accomplishment was as a physician for which he achieved so much respect and acclaim that he was declared the god of healing two thousand years after he died. His tomb became a shrine comparable to modern Lourdes in France where people come today in search of cures.[1] His work as a healer became so widely known that scholars traveled to Egypt to learn his methods. Greek philosophers **Thales** (624-546 B.C.), **Anaximander** (610-546 B.C.), **Pythagoras** (560-480 B.C.), **Democritus** (470-380 B.C.), and the famous Greek traveler **Hecataeus** (550-476 B.C.) all visited Egypt.

According to **Herodotus** (c.484-c.424 B.C.), a world-class traveler and historian, Egyptian doctors practiced in only one disease or specialty. Some specialized in diseases of the eye, others of the head, others of the teeth, others of the stomach and organs around the belly. Some dealt with troubles that could not be identified easily, in other words, internal medicine. Herodotus described the health routine of Egyptian farmers. They purged themselves every month for three successive days, and they used emetics and enemas to further preserve their health. They believed that all diseases were related to their diet.[2]

Shen Nung was a god of medicine in China, where the concept of *Yin* and *Yang* became a doctrine of healing several thousand years ago. The original philosophy of yin and yang was that there are two opposing elements of the universe—male and female. Yin is the female principle and element of the universe standing for darkness, cold, and death. Yang is the male principle and element of the universe, the source of life and heat, and with Yin, co-creator of everything that is. The idea of yin and yang has been so modified by blending with the thoughts of various religions that the original philosophy becomes incomprehensible.

Inevitably, the power of religion played a major role in healing. **Moses**, who led the Israelites out of Egypt and received the ten commandments from god, drew up a sanitation and diet code for the Hebrews that had the force of religious doctrine.

MESOPOTAMIA

From the mountains of Turkey and the elevated hills of Armenia two great rivers rise, the Euphrates and the Tigris, which flow in devious courses toward the south and come together where they enter the Persian Gulf. The country at the upper region of the Tigris was called Assyria and the region near the southern part of the Euphrates was called Babylonia. The southern portion of the two rivers was a low plain built up over time by a rich river mud. The climate was, and is, hot and dry. The land to the north above Baghdad is fertile plateau more moderate in temperature and with some rainfall. The region to the west of the Euphrates extending to the Mediterranean consists largely of the area known as Syria.[3]

The Greeks gave the name Mesopotamia to the long, narrow stretch of land between the Tigris and Euphrates rivers. In Greek, *mesopotamia* means *between the rivers*. The land is now part of Iraq. Settlers lived in Mesopotamia before 4000 B.C. No one knows where they came from, their language or race. Later inhabitants included the Sumerians and Semites.

The Sumerians who may have migrated from the mountainous regions of Turkey and Iran developed a remarkably advanced civilization after 3000 B.C. They had knowledge of mathematics, astronomy, and medicine. They devised the 360-degree circle and the 60 minute hour. They built palaces and temples in their cities and their craftsmen worked in gold, copper, silver and stone. They wove cloth, made swords, spears, armor, and chariots for their armies.[5]

The economy of Sumer was based on agriculture involving several kinds of crops. They built a system of irrigation canals for growing barley, wheat, date palms, and vegetables. They used domestic animals such as sheep, goats, and donkeys. Their settlements grew into cities and city-states, and by armed takeover into small kingdoms.

They invented a form of writing, called *cuneiform* in which wedge shaped figures were punched into clay with a stylus. The cuneiform writing was the standard form of writing and keeping records. The method was adopted by other people and used for centuries. Thousands of these clay tablets have been discovered and preserved. They tell about the government, law, business practices, and religion of the Sumerians. The widespread use of the cuneiform method of record keeping and communicating reminds one of the practice in recent times called *lingua franca*, a hybrid language of Italian, Spanish, French, Greek, Arabic, and Turkish elements that was spoken initially at Mediterranean ports and eventually for communicating among different nationalities.

The oldest medical treatise known was on a clay tablet 3¾ by 6¼ inches written by a Sumerian physician who collected and recorded more than a dozen of his favorite remedies and prescriptions for his students and colleagues. It lay buried in the ruins for more than 4000 years before being excavated by an American expedition and brought to the University Museum in Philadelphia. The Sumerian physician leaned on botanical, mineral, and zoological material. His favorite mineral was sodium chloride (salt) and potassium nitrate (saltpeter). From animal sources he used milk, snake skin, and turtle shell. Most of his medicines were botanical: Cassia, myrtle, asafoetida, and thyme as well as products from trees such as pear, fig, fir, and date. Medicines were prepared from seed, root, branch, bark or gum. Some of the remedies were to be taken internally and some were for external application, including salves. The compounding of salves was to pulverize the materials and infuse the powder with a wine and mix it with a vegetable oil such as cedar oil. If the pulverized material contained clay the powder was mixed with water and honey. For remedies to be taken internally, beer was the standby to make them palatable. Sometimes milk was used instead of beer, or with it.

Our anonymous physician never mentioned diseases that the remedies were for, nor the amount of a remedy to make a dose. But there was much speculation about the causes of diseases. Like physicians of later times, they talked about demons, gods, and goddesses but pinning down a cause didn't arrive until several millennia later.[6]

By 2000 B.C. the Sumerians lost their political power to the invading Semites who set the stage for the Babylonian civilization.

In Babylonia there were two classes of specialists who dealt with diseases. The *ashipu* practiced magic, and the *asu* were physicians who prescribed practical remedies. Hundreds of diseases were recognized. Physicians in Babylonia were rigidly controlled, as were most trades and services by a set of laws called *The Code of Hammurabi*. **Hammurabi** ruled the Babylonian empire with an iron fist for 43 years (about 1792 to about 1750 B.C.) during which he revised and expanded laws in effect since 300 years earlier. Under the Code, physician's fees were stipulated, the amount depending on the kind and extent of treatment. Stiff penalties were imposed for failure to heal, usually involving a painfully physical disfigurement. Prisons were not suitable punishment in Babylonia. Physical punishment was quicker, cheaper, and more effective as a deterrent. For example, if a couple was found guilty of adultery, the man was castrated and the woman's nose cut off. Babylonia was not a healthy place for healers suspected of misconduct or quackery.

The principal of physical retaliation in which even accidental death or mutilation was required in kind was probably a holdover from earlier, more brutal times. There were differences in penalties and privileges that depended on the social class of the individual. If a physician saved the life of a patient with what was considered appropriate treatment he was given a handsome reward. If a patient died following what was thought to be bad practice, he would have a hand cut off. Penalties and rewards were a mixture of primitive practice and more liberal thinking. A slave had the right to marry a free woman and to beget free children. In a remarkably liberal feature of the code not ordinarily experienced for thousands of years later, a widow had the right to own property and conduct a business in her name.[7]

We get a quick view of the health status of the people of Mesopotamia from excavations of burial sites. At a site called Chatal Huyuk, "Judging from the bones, the people were fairly healthy, though many were anemic, possibly as a result of malaria, and others suffered from arthritis or limb fractures. On average, men lived to the age of 34 and women to 30."

King **Sennacherib** (704-681 BC) built a palace in Nineveh but became engaged in bitter warfare at the end of which Babylon had to surrender to the Assyrians. Sennacherib's retaliation was harsh. He carried away the city's wealth, smashed the temples, palaces, and statues of the gods, and destroyed the houses. Some of the debris was dumped into the Euphrates and carried away. Sennacherib was assassinated by one of his sons, and another son, **Esarhaddon** (680-669 BC) was named crown prince. The gods **Shamash** and **Adad** were consulted by oracles and Esarhaddon was made king. But he was not in good health. He complained of fever, weakness, loss of appetite, stiff joints, eye infections, earache, chills, and skin problems. He was treated with lotions, ointments, rest, change of diet, and religious rituals. It was all to no avail, and this gave him bouts of depression. Diseases, it was widely believed, were from the actions of gods. Esarhaddon wondered what the gods wanted of him. Before he became King, court astrologers had reported on omens from the stars. Mercury, the star of the crown prince, was in conjunction with Saturn, the star of the king, on 18 May 681 BC. This was interpreted as predicting the murder of the king and the restoration of the temples by his successor. Therefore, Esarhaddon reversed his father's actions and ordered the temples of Babylon rebuilt. Presumably, it made him feel better.[8]

CHAPTER 2

HIPPOCRATES

In Greek culture the god of medicine was **Asclepias**, a healer so renowned that, according to Greek mythology, **Zeus** slew him with a thunderbolt for daring to bring a man back to life, thus threatening the gods' monopoly on immortality. The temple of Asclepias was where physicians, called **Asclepiads**, practiced under the influence of priests who taught that recovery of their patients depended on the will of the gods, **Hygieia** and **Panacea**. Hygieia was a version of **Athena**, the goddess of reason who was concerned with prevention of disease and maintaining health. Panacea was the god who specialized in drugs. The word *panacea* in our vocabulary refers to the idea that a medicine can solve all health problems.[1, 2, 3]

There came on the scene a man with new ways of healing so insightful and sound that the influence of his ideas and methods of practice permeates the medical profession even today. **Hippocrates** is called the father of modern medicine. He rejected dependence on the gods of the temple. He prescribed rest and relaxation to permit the natural power of the body to heal itself. He prescribed drugs sparingly, and surgery rarely, only as a last resort. Health spas were set up in locations having beautiful surroundings near mountain springs or on the sunny shores of the Aegean Sea where the patient was free of the routine anxieties of life, given hydrotherapy, cleansing baths, ointments, abstinence, a healthful diet, and a contemplative atmosphere.

Hippocrates was born on the Aegean island of Cos about 460 B.C. Little is known about his early background. Tradition has it that he was born into a family descended from Asclepias. Tradition has it that Hippocrates visited Egypt early in life and there studied the healing methods of Imhotep. He practiced in Athens where he is credited with bringing a "plague", possibly smallpox, under control, but eventually he returned to the healing center at Cos where he founded a school to teach his method of healing devoid of superstitions and religious incantations. He laid down principles of treatment that placed responsibility for curing squarely on the shoulders of the physician.

Students were required to agree to principles of professional practice, many of which survive in today's medical schools, where a revised version of the Hippocratic Oath is recited by graduating students.

The Oath was and is a binding code of ethics. While not risking the disfavor of the gods, the Oath says:

I swear by Apollo the healer, by Asclepias, by Health and all the powers of healing, and call to witness all the gods and goddesses that I may keep this oath.

I will pay the same respect to my teacher as to my parents. I will regard his sons as my brothers and teach them the science (medicine) if they desire to learn it, without fee or contract. I will pass on precepts, lectures and all other learning to my sons, to those of my teacher and to those pupils duly apprenticed and sworn, and to none other.

I will use my power to help the sick to the best of my ability and judgment. I will abstain from harming or wronging any man by it.

I will not give a fatal draught to anyone if I am asked, nor will I suggest any such a thing. Neither will I give a woman means to obtain an abortion.

I will be chaste and religious in my life and in my practice.

I will not cut, even for the stone, but will leave such procedures to the practitioners of that craft.

Whenever I go into a house, it will be to help the sick and never to do any harm or injury. I will not abuse my position to indulge in sexual contacts with women or men, whether they be freemen or slaves.

Whatever I see or hear, professionally or privately, that ought not to be divulged, I will keep secret and tell no one.

If I observe this oath and do not violate it, may I prosper both in my life and in my profession, earning good repute among all men for all time. If I transgress and forswear this Oath, may my lot be otherwise.

The Hippocratic Oath is not the only tradition to survive the millennia of time to be honored in today's medical practice. The symbol of the art and science of medicine and healing is called the *caduceus*, consisting of a winged staff entwined with two serpents. The staff with wings represents

Mercury, the messenger god with wings on his hat. The serpents have special meaning. Since early times, serpents have been thought of as representing either good or evil. The Bible tells how the subtle serpent persuaded **Eve** to eat the forbidden fruit, and then the woman encouraged **Adam** to eat the fruit as well. Adam and Eve were banned from Eden and thereafter had to making a living in agriculture. The good side of the serpent is the act of shedding its old skin every year and emerging with a bright new one which is seen as a process of renewal and rejuvenation. Thus the serpents on the caduceus symbolize the performance of physicians in restoring health and prevailing over death.

Today the caduceus is used to adorn printed material or portrayed on the outer walls of medical buildings as a sign of their purpose. The caduceus is placed on the sleeves and shirt collars of army and navy medical officers to distinguish them from line officers.

Another link between the Hippocratic Oath and today's medical practice is that the Oath is clearly the statement of a guild: powerful, exclusive, protecting its secrets. One might see in some respects a resemblance to the AMA (American Medical Association): powerful and exclusive. The habit of some doctors of writing prescriptions that are illegible to anyone but doctors and pharmacists seems like a survival of earlier times.

More than fifty books comprise what is called the *Hippocratic Corpus*, believed to have been written by many authors between 420 and 370 B.C. It is impossible to tell which of the books were actually written by Hippocrates. No doubt many of the authors were former students. They give an account of Hippocrates' methods that included determining the patient's history, close observations of symptoms, documentation of the patients response to treatment, and detailed descriptions of the onset, prognosis and outcome of many diseases. They believed in cleanliness for both patient and physician, ample rest for the sick or impaired, and above all, that the physician should let nature take its course in the healing process.

Some of the writings describe the use of drugs. Most were of doubtful benefit. We find reference to hellebore (a plant that has pesticide properties) to induce vomiting, cantharides (blister beetles powdered or soaked) for dropsy, squill and other botanicals, and some minerals for various ailments. Used, but rarely, were aggressive treatments such as purges and bleeding.

The main focus of the physicians of the Hippocratic school was the master's teaching that nature should be allowed to pursue the healing process: "Our natures are the physicians of our diseases."

Hippocratic medicine flourished during the latter part of the golden age of Greece that peaked in the fifth century BC, during the time of great philosophers and scientists such as **Thales** of Miletus (624-546 BC) regarded by later Greeks as the founder of Greek science, mathematics and philosophy, **Pythagoras** of Samos and Croton in southern Italy (about 560-480 BC) who is supposed to have coined the word "philosopher", and **Alcmaeon** (born in Croton about 535 B.C) a Greek physician who was the first person on record to have conducted dissections of the human body. They were followed by equally great philosopher-scientists: **Democritus** (about 470-380 BC) best known for his atomic theory of matter, **Socrates** (470-399 BC), a brave soldier and disciplined philosopher, his chief disciple, **Plato** (427-347 BC), who was preeminently a moral philosopher, and **Aristotle** (384-322 BC) who was a pupil of Plato and became the most renowned thinker and natural scientist of ancient Greece.

It was a time of great intellectual creativity but it was also a time of political turmoil. Animosity between Athens and Sparta resulted in the disastrous Peloponnesian wars. They slugged it out from 431 to 377 BC, leaving the Greek city states so exhausted that they were attractive targets for the ambitions of **Philip II** (382-336) of Macedon who defeated the combined armies of Athens and Thebes in 338 BC. The decisive battle was a cavalry charge led by Philip's brash 18 year-old son, **Alexander**. Shortly after his father's death, the 20 year-old **Alexander the Great** (356-323 B.C.) embarked on his campaign to conquer the world.

Even when very young, Alexander was ambitious. When he heard of Philip's conquests he wept and complained, "My father will get ahead of me in everything and will leave nothing great for me to do." As a boy he was fearless and strong. He tamed a spirited horse named Bucephala that no one else dared to touch or ride. During Alexander's conquest the horse carried him all the way to India where it died.

When Alexander was 14 years old his father employed Aristotle as his teacher. Alexander was eager to learn. Under his tutor he acquired a love of literature. He came to know and like Greek ways and ideals and Greek civilization. Aristotle inspired Alexander to take an interest in other countries and races of people, and also taught him of animals and plants.

The greatest thinker of ancient times influenced the young man destined to become the greatest soldier of ancient times in many beneficial ways but there is no indication that he had any influence on the young man's ambition to conquer the world. Aristotle's nephew, **Callisthenes**, who accompanied Alexander on his campaign, was executed during a drunken rage by the obsessively ambitious conqueror. Among other accomplishments, Alexander founded the city of Alexandria in Egypt. It was there that one of his generals, **Ptolemy** (367-283 B.C.), who acquired the rule of Egypt, founded the famous Alexandrian library and museum that became the preeminent world seat of learning. The *Hippocratic Corpus* was gathered there about 250 BC.

Hippocrates' methods flourished in Greek medical practice for 500 years after his death, or until about AD 370, after which healers of many persuasions reverted to less enlightened practices. While Rome had become the unquestioned seat of power throughout the region, Greek physicians were still recognized as the preeminent healers.[4]

CHAPTER 3

GALEN

Followers of Hippocrates were still in full bloom when there appeared on the scene a luminary called **Galen** whose words on healing were gospel that would dominate the practice of medicine in Western Europe for more than a millennium. In 1559, thirteen centuries after Galen's death, a member of the College of Physicians in London is said to have been forced to recant for having the temerity to question Galen's work.

Galen was born in Pergamum (now Bergama in Turkey) about 130 AD and died, probably in Sicily, about 200 AD. Tradition has it that his father, who was a wealthy architect, had a dream in which **Asclepias**, the Greek god of medicine, came to him and said, "Make a physician of your son." Young Galen made his father's dream come true. He obtained an education by spending his youthful years traveling around the eastern provinces of the Roman Empire during which he visited and apparently attended the prestigious medical school in Alexandria. At the age of 29 he was appointed physician to the gladiatorial school at Pergamum which gave him raw experience and observation of human anatomy. Two years later he went to Rome where he spent most of his professional life.

Galen's greatest contribution was as a pioneer in the study of anatomy, building on his experience with gladiators. It was not considered proper at that time to experiment on human bodies, so he restricted his exploratory work to dissections of animals including dogs, goats, pigs, and monkeys. He wrote extensively and described his work in detail, but his observations were not always applicable to humans. In a study of the heart he deduced that the blood had to get from the one side of the heart to the other and that there must be tiny holes through which the blood flowed. It was not until 14 centuries later that an English physician, **William Harvey** (1578-

1657), determined the true function of the heart and the circulation of the blood. However, Galen's best work was with muscles in which he showed how they worked in combinations. He did more than observe; he experimented. For example, in one of his studies with live animals he severed the spinal cord at different levels and noted the parts of the body that were affected by paralysis. He carefully described a network of blood vessels under the brain, present in many animals but not in man, but Galen assigned it an important role in the functioning of the human body. However he did especially good work on muscles, probably derived from his experiences on gladiators, describing in detail for the first time the functions of various muscles. He was the first to use the pulse as a diagnostic aid, and he described the flow of urine through the uterus to the bladder.

Galen was a prolific writer, leaving many of his opinions and observations for medical professionals to use as guides for their practices. He engaged in polemics with other physicians and was adamant in his opinions. He was arrogant, disputatious, and pompous in self esteem. He saw little of value in the teachings and practice of Hippocrates. He was emphatic in being anti-atomist.

The Greek philosopher **Democritus** (460 B.C.-370 B.C.) maintained that the Milky Way was a vast conglomerate of tiny stars, and that the moon was an earthlike world with mountains and valleys. He is best known for his atomic theory. He believed that all matter consisted of tiny particles, almost infinitely small, so small that nothing smaller is conceivable. Thus, they were indivisible. The word "atom" means "indivisible." The atoms, he held, were eternal, unchangeable, indestructible. Besides the atoms themselves, only the void—that is the space between them—existed.

Galen, by rejecting the theory of atoms missed out on perpetuating an idea of matter that is gospel today. Galen's lack was in understanding physiology, having adopted the "humors" theory of disease, that is, that disease is caused by an imbalance of the vital fluids, or humors, of the body, an idea first advanced by the philosopher Empedocles (c. 492-c. 432 BC). The humors theory remained popular for centuries, eventually becoming four in number: blood, phlegm, black bile, and yellow bile.

Galen engaged in heated arguments with other physicians to whom he was known as an arrogant braggart. His unpopularity in professional circles eventually drove him back to his home in Pergamum but his reputation with the fashionable clientele in Rome did not escape the attention of emperor, **Marcus Aurelius** (AD 161-188), who called him back to be court physician. Galen was also employed by emperors **Commodius** (180-192) and **Septimius Severus** (193-211). The reign of Marcus Aurelius, best known for his writings, notably his *Meditations*, was during the latter part of the most majestic days of the Roman Empire which at the death of **Trajan** in AD 117 extended from the shores of the Caspian Sea and the Persian Gulf on the east to the Atlantic Coast of Spain on the west, and from Britain in the north to Egypt in the south. In short, the Roman Empire encompassed what was seen then as the entire civilized western world.

Many of Galen's views might have been discarded except for a quirk of history. Contrary to the prevailing views of Greeks and Romans about gods and goddesses, Galen leaned toward monotheism. Although not a Christian himself, he believed that everything in the universe was made by God for a purpose and that there was a design in everything including the human body. The idea appealed to both Christians and Muslims. It made certain that his books would remain popular with physicians through the Middle Ages.[2]

CHAPTER 4

HEALERS OF THE MIDDLE AGES

In defiance of stagnation in medical advances since the early Greek healers of the Hippocrates and Galen schools, there appeared a Swiss alchemist and physician who called himself **Paracelsus** (1493-1541). Born in Einsiedein (the year after Columbus discovered the Americas), Paracelsus' real name was **Philippus Aureolus Theophrastus Bombastus von Hohenheim**, but in a vainglorious splurge gave himself the name Paracelsus, meaning "better than" or "equal to" **Celsus**, a Roman encyclopedist born about 10 BC who wrote eight books in Latin on Greek knowledge and learning. The only writings of Celsus that survived were his detailed descriptions of medical practice, which in the exaggerated interpretation of later times gave Celsus the reputation of an exceptionally competent physician. His writing was lost in the Middle Ages but was rediscovered in 1426 and printed in 1478 when physicians of the Renaissance were eager for what they thought must be the most reliable medical knowledge available. Paracelsus had a flamboyant, contentious personality whose mentality was a conglomerate of sound thinking, suppositions, gullibility, and absurdity. He ridiculed the theory of humours but espoused the four elements proposed by the Greeks and believed that there were the three basic principles: mercury, sulfur and salt. He believed in the influence of the stars on disease and he engaged in a search for the philosopher's stone, insisting that if he could find it he would live forever. He became the town surgeon of Basel and a professor of medicine which enabled him to lecture to the faculty of the medical school. He lectured in German instead of the customary Latin and wore the rustic leather apron of an alchemist. Although, like most physicians of the time, he was contemptuous of surgeons for using their hands instead of their minds for healing, he allowed the barber surgeons to attend his classes. In a remarkably enlightened view of mental illness; he scoffed at the idea that people could be possessed of demons.

One way of looking at Paracelsus' work is that he promoted the transition of alchemy to chemistry and medicine, for he concluded that the purpose of alchemy was not to find ways of converting other materials into gold but to make medicines. Most of the reliable medicines up to that time were botanicals but in Paracelsus' view, minerals were an overlooked resource. His favorites were compounds of mercury and antimony but he also subscribed to iron, arsenic, lead, copper, and sulfur. His vigorous promotion of minerals for treating diseases, although widely condemned, appealed to some respected physicians.

Paracelsus' greatest impact on the practice of medicine, aside from inciting controversy and therefore a new wave of more modern thinking in the treatment of diseases, was the widespread adoption of toxic minerals as medicines, the indiscriminate and dangerous use of which continued for 400 years, with lingering use into the present, a topic that will be mentioned later in a discussion of vaccines. But things were beginning to happen in science generally.

Meanwhile, though progress in methods of healing had lagged in Europe through the centuries, Arabic scholars wrote volumes of texts on medical topics. The most prolific was the Persian physician **Avicenna** (980-1037) whose full name was Abu al-Husayn ibn Abdallah ibn Sina. He was born near Bukhara in what is now Uzbek and died in Hamadan in what is now northwest Iran. Avicenna, regarded as the greatest physician of medieval times, was an infant genius who could recite the entire Koran by heart at the age of 10 and was practicing medicine when he was 16. A prodigious worker, he is credited with writing more than 250 books including two encyclopedias, one on science and another on medicine, the *Kitab al Qanun* (*Canon*, or Medical Code), consisting of five books: I General principles, II Descriptions of simple drugs (lists 760 drugs separately), III Specific diseases, IV Diseases of the whole body including poisons, and V Compound drugs and their uses. He wrote at least forty other books on medicine. Avicenna's ideas were based largely on the theories and work of Hippocrates and Galen. There was little innovation beyond the methods of the Greek physicians although Avicenna's detailed descriptions of surgical procedures is evidence of significant advances in surgery. When Avicenna's work was translated into Latin in the twelfth century, the *Canon* became the most authoritative medical textbook in use, and remained popular until the beginning of the Scientific Revolution, or about 1600. And, it is said to still have an influence on medical practice in Islamic parts of the world.

Another Persian physician-philosopher and prolific writer was **Muhammad ibn Zakariya al-Razi**, known to westerners as **Rhazes** (865-925) whose influence on medical thinking still flourished 500 years after his death. He left about 200 writings of which the most popular of his work was translated into Latin and reprinted several times for physicians of the Latin West between 1488 and 1542.

The chaotic state of medications during medieval times is seen in *Kitab al-sumum* (*Book on Poisons*) by **Abu Bakr M. b. 'Ali b. Wahshiya al-Nabati** also called **Ibn Wahshiya**, born of Aramaic or Syriac parents in Iraq during the ninth century A.D. As a Nabatean, he bragged about his ancestors being of a high culture, and though a Muslim, he despised the Arabs as an inferior people. The *Book on Poisons* is probably the first comprehensive study of the toxicology of drugs. It is a detailed discussion of poisons and their antidotes. The Middle Ages were politically fluid times in which intrigue, assassination and its ever present threat were tools of high level, power-hungry schemers. Members of the Italian Borgia family, prominent in the 1400's and 1500's, were classic examples of treachery and wickedness in which poisons were often the road to success. Ibn Wahshiya worked both sides of the street. His book contains detailed instructions for the preparation of a stunning array of poisons and, for each, the antidote. Poisons for the most part were well known plant poisons, minerals, and some derived from insects and other animals. Antidotes were mostly complicated concoctions of bizarre ingredients, sometimes requiring elaborate preparation. None of them would find a place in today's *Physician's Desk Reference*.

PART II
THE SCIENTIFIC REVOLUTION

5 SEEING THE UNSEEABLE

6 HEART AND BLOOD

7 PASTEUR

8 THE EXPLORER

9 THE IMMUNIZERS

10 PASTEUR'S VACCINATION

11 PEAS AND PEOPLE

CHAPTER 5

SEEING THE UNSEEABLE

The microscope is to health and healing what the telescope is to astronomy and exploration of the universe. Discovery of microbes opened the window to a new understanding of diseases and how to cope with their causes and cures. There was a thriving industry of lens grinding and spectacle making during the sixteenth century in Europe. The most advanced lens makers were in the Netherlands. One of them, **Zacharias Janssen** (1580-1638), reasoned that if one lens would magnify things two lenses would magnify even more. So in 1590 he put a convex lens at each end of a tube and found that magnification was indeed increased. It was the first microscope. In a related innovation **Hans Lippershey** (1570-1619), a German-Dutch lens grinder and spectacles maker, had an apprentice who while idly handling lenses, held two of them before his eyes and noticed that it made distant things seem closer and larger (and upside down). He told his boss about it and Lippershey was astounded. He made a telescope by mounting two lenses on opposite ends of a tube and offered to sell the invention to the Dutch government, which at the time was engaged in a war of rebellion against Spain. The government made an effort to keep the invention a military secret, but without success. Rumors of it reached **Galileo** (1564-1642) who made a telescope of his own, one that had the power to magnify 32 times and would enable him to see the four major moons of Jupiter. He also arranged the lenses in reverse, producing an improved microscope.[1,2]

Johann Kepler (1571-1630), a German astronomer who taught science at the University of Graz in Austria, then at Prague, obtained one of the telescopes that Galileo made and devised an improvement. He also described, in theory, a microscope that would be better than any then available. Further improvement, in which others participated, led to the compound microscope, an instrument that revolutionized findings in biology and medicine.

An English physicist, **Robert Hooke** (1635-1701), took up the use of the microscope and became one of the greatest of the early microscopists. His work, *Micrographia*, published in 1665, displays some of the most beautiful drawings ever made of microscopic objects. The observation of which he is most famous, was on the structure of cork. A thin slice of cork viewed under the microscope showed a mass of compact rectangular holes. He called them *cells*, from a Latin word meaning "small chamber," especially like those in rows as in prison cells. Because cork is dead tissue consisting of bark of the cork tree, it was not evident at the time that there was any relation between Hooke's "cells" and the cells we see in living tissue, but the name stuck.

The first person to actually see living things that were too small to be seen with the naked eye was a Dutch microscopist, **Antoni van Leeuwenhoek** (1631-1723). In 1676, using a microscope with a small, single lens that he had ground to perfection, he put a sample of pond water under the lens and saw what he called *animalcules* of various kinds. The modern term is *microorganisms*. In 1677, he observed spermatozoa in semen. Later, in 1683, he saw objects so small that they were barely detectable under the lens. He thought they must be living organisms. No one else had been able to produce such finely ground lenses, and it would be another century before anyone would be able to confirm that what Leeuwenhoek had seen were probably bacteria. The discovery of microorganisms was destined to put the study of health and disease on a new level. Leeuwenhoek's finding was the foundation for *bacteriology* as a special branch of science under a German botanist, **Ferdinand Julius Cohn** (1828-1898). The new science was a stepping stone for proving the validity of the revolutionary "germ theory of disease." (see Pasteur, chapter 7). The science was expanded to what is now called *microbiology* which includes all microscopic and submicroscopic organisms. There followed a parade of discoveries related to the role of microorganisms in the cause of diseases, and their treatment.

A major advance in the study of bacteria was a method of staining them. When in 1884 a Danish bacteriologist, **Hans Christian Joachim Gram** (1853-1938) stained some bacteria with a dye and treated them with iodine then washed them with alcohol. The procedure would remove the stain from some kinds of bacteria but not from others. Bacteriologists called the bacteria that retained the dye *Gram-positive* and bacteria that lost the dye *Gram-negative*. It was found that the two types of bacteria differ in their susceptibility to anti-bacterials. Some bactericides are effective against Gram-positive bacteria and others are effective against Gram-negative bacteria. This is obviously important to know when you're treating an infection.

A major advance in the study of microorganisms was the development of the electron microscope. Given the sophistication that had been built into microscopes with carefully ground lenses and optical systems, there was still the need for more magnification to study microorganisms and their physical features, and to find and study organisms of smaller size. A limitation of ordinary light microscopes is that if the object is smaller than half the wavelength of light, it cannot be seen because the light will simply go around it. An object has to cast a shadow to be seen. Therefore, a shorter wavelength than that of visible light would make it possible to detect smaller objects and more detailed features.[3]

It had been known for a long time that electromagnetic radiation, which includes light and X rays, has both particle and wave aspects. It was found, too, that an electron beam had wave properties. Thus, reasoned **Ernest August Friedrich Ruska** (1906-1988), a German electrical engineer, it should be possible to manipulate a beam of electrons as a beam of light, and to focus it on objects.[4] Electrons cannot be focused through a lens but since they are electrically charged they can be focused by using magnetic fields. Electrons have wavelengths much shorter than visible light or X rays. Since the shorter the wavelength, the smaller the objects that can be detected and the sharper the focus, an electron microscope should be much more powerful than an ordinary light microscope.

In 1932, Ruska and a collaborator, **Max Knoll**, built the first such instrument. Although a crude experimental design, it would magnify 400 times, about twice that of a good ordinary light microscope. A Canadian-American physicist, **James Hillier**, and his collaborator, **Albert P. Prebus**, built an improved model in 1937 that would magnify 7,000 times. Further improvements were made in the instruments, some of them magnifying 2,000,000 times, making visible fine details down to the size of large molecules.[5]

Ruska, for his pioneering contribution was awarded the Nobel Prize for physics in 1986.

CHAPTER 6

SOLVING THE MYSTERY OF THE HEART AND BLOOD

Galen, a Greek physician of the second century AD, had recognized that there was circulation of the blood and surmised that there were pores in the wall between the ventricles of the heart that permitted the blood to flow from one side to the other. Ten centuries later, an Arabic scholar, **Ibn al-Nafis** (d. 1288), wrote a book in 1242 in which he proposed that the right and left ventricles were completely separate and that the right ventricle pumped blood through arteries that led to the lungs where progressively smaller vessels picked up blood from the lungs. These small vessels led into larger vessels that led back to the left ventricle, and that pumped the blood out to the body. Thus, Al-Nafis hit on the functioning of the heart and lungs in the circulation of the blood, called the *lesser circulation*. But his book was not known to the West until 1942, so it had no effect on subsequent work.[1]

A Spanish physician, **Miguel Servet**, better known as **Michael Servetus** (1511-1553), described the lesser circulation of the blood in a book which, however, was mainly devoted to his theological views as a Unitarian. While seeking refuge for his religious life, he made the mistake of venturing into Geneva which at the time was under the control of **John Calvin**, a strict Presbyterian reformer and deadly enemy of anyone deviating in the slightest degree from his precepts. Calvin declared and defined in detail "immoral practices" which included most forms of fun and entertainment. Servetus was arrested, tried as a heretic, and burned at the stake. Calvin attempted to burn all copies of Servetus's book, but some unburned copies were found in 1694.

An Italian anatomist, **Realdo Colombo** (c.1510-1559) in 1559 wrote a detailed and thorough account of the lesser circulation and his was the first work to come to the attention of the medical profession, so he is credited with the discovery of the lesser circulation. But still it remained for another to determine and to describe the full circulatory system of the blood.[2]

The first person to fully trace the circulation of the blood through the body was **William Harvey** (1578-1657), an English physician. Harvey took his university degree at Cambridge and studied at the medical school in Padua, Italy. While there, he may have been inspired by the brilliance of **Galileo** (1564-1642) whose passion for experimentation Harvey also possessed. Returning to England, he engaged in a successful career as a physician, becoming court physician to **James I** (1566-1625), son of **Mary**, Queen of Scots, and to James' son **Charles I** (1600-1649) who apparently stayed healthy until rebellion broke out under the leadership of **Oliver Cromwell** (1599-1658) during which Charles fled to Scotland. But the Scottish leaders handed him over to Parliament. He was convicted of treason and beheaded in 1649.

Harvey's finding on blood circulation was published in 1616 under the title *Exercitatio de Motu Cordis et Sanguinis* (On the Motions of the Heart and Blood). It was a classic report on careful scientific experiments and observations, but his conclusions were met with sarcastic criticism by those who cited the second century Greek physician, **Galen** (about 130-200), as the supposedly irrefutable authority. They called him Harvey "the Circulator," a name used for peddlers of medicines at the circus, actually Latin slang for quack.

While in medical school at Padua, Harvey had studied under the Italian physician **Girolamo Fabrici** (1537-1619), better known by his Latinized name, **Fabricius ab Aquapendente**, who had discovered the one-way valves in the veins, which he described in a book in 1603. He pointed out that blood was pumped by muscular action through the veins toward the heart and that the valves kept the blood from flowing back. But Fabrici either did not recognize their significance or did not dare to refute the centuries-old claims of Galen. Harvey's finding was that the blood is pumped out of the right ventricle, goes to the lungs, returns to the left ventricle which pumps it through arteries to all parts of the body, from where it returns to the right ventricle through the veins. Although Harvey traced both the arteries and veins separately only to their visible limits, which did not include the microscopic capillaries, his experiments and reasoned conclusions about the function of the heart and blood circulation convinced him that the arteries and veins were connected. He was right, but was not proved correct until **Marcello Malpighi** (1628-1694), an Italian physiologist and physician whom some have called the father of microscopy, observed the capillaries under his microscope.

Thus it became clear that Harvey's findings would demolish the centuries-old addiction of his fellow physicians to Galen's antiquated medicine. Harvey came to be respected and honored by most of his former critics. He is now regarded as the founder of modern physiology.[3]

Further understanding of the role of blood came when **Jan Swammerdam** (1637-1680), a Dutch naturalist, announced in 1658 the discovery of red blood corpuscles. Although Swammerdam had obtained a medical degree from Leiden University, he never practiced it. During his short life he collected some three thousand specimens of insects, and using a microscope that had been greatly improved during the fifty years since Janssen's invention, he produced studies of insect microanatomy, including the way muscles change shape during contraction, and he detailed the reproductive organs of insects. But he is most remembered for discovering the red corpuscles. The blood stream contains billions of the corpuscles but it was not known until later that their function is to carry oxygen from the lungs to tissues throughout the body.

CHAPTER 7

PASTEUR

Louis Pasteur (1822-1895), whose name is remembered by most people for pasteurization of milk and other mostly liquid foods, was a scientist of remarkable accomplishments. He was among the most prolific of scientific investigators and probably the greatest contributor of all time to health and healing. **Isaac Asimov**, eminent writer and science historian, said of Pasteur, "…recognized both in his lifetime and ever since as one of the greatest scientist in history. In biology it is doubtful that anyone but Aristotle and Darwin can be mentioned in the same breath with him."

Pasteur was born in Dôle, a small town in eastern France. His parents encouraged him to pursue studies toward a professional career, but as a youth Pasteur was not an outstanding student. He did fairly well in mathematics, and received a grade of "mediocre" in chemistry. He was more interested in painting for which he had considerable talent. He had started painting portraits while in his early teens and he wanted to make art his life's work, hopefully becoming a teacher of fine arts. He did tutoring to sustain himself, and like many aspiring artists he struggled against poverty bordering on starvation. But events changed his life, and fortunately, the welfare of mankind.

Pasteur attended lectures of the prominent chemists, **Jean Baptiste André Dumas** and **Antoine Jérôme Balard**, who so inspired him that he decided to pursue chemistry as a profession. He had studied for the entrance examination to the Ecole Normale Supérieure, an elite school in Paris for students headed for professional work in literature, arts, and sciences. He passed the examination and was admitted, in 1842, with the rank of sixteenth. But, disappointed in not ranking in the top tier, he turned down the appointment and decided to spend more time studying for a repeat of the exam. The attention to detail in his painting may have honed his innate passion for perfection that pervaded his career. In the following year he took the examination again and passed with a rank of fifth.

RIGHT HANDED AND LEFT HANDED CRYSTALS

Having established a background in physics and chemistry, in 1847, Pasteur at the age of twenty four, continued at the École Normale Supérieure on research for his doctor's degree. He decided to study crystals. It was a choice in which he could hardly go wrong because crystallography was a popular subject at the École Normale where one of the professors had done work on quartz crystals. So it was already known in Pasteur's time that polarized light passing through quartz would change its direction. Many organic substances, either liquids or solids in solution, had a curious effect on light. Polarized light (screened to produce light rays in only one direction) passing through them would be twisted to the right or left.

Pasteur was intrigued. There was an interest in tartrates, possibly because tartaric acid is an important constituent of wine, forming the "tarter" during fermentation. In 1848 he made crystals of a salt of tartaric acid (ammonium sodium tartrate). He examined the crystals under a microscope and noted that they differed in appearance, some facing left and some facing right. He meticulously separated the right and left facing crystals with tweezers and determined that one kind twisted polarized light to the right and the other kind twisted light to the left although both had been crystallized from the same solution. When he dissolved the right- and left-handed crystals in separate containers, the solutions twisted light only in the same direction as their respective crystals, called dextrorotatory (right) and levorotatory (left). The letters *d-* and *l-* are used to designate these characteristics, or simply (+) and (-). Another way to designate right or left configuration is with R (rectus) or S (sinistral).

There was also a so-called third form of tartrate, of the same chemical composition, that did not polarize light. As Pasteur suspected, when he dissolved the two kinds of crystals together, the solution did not rotate the plane of polarized light because the effect of one kind of crystal was neutralized by the counter effect of its mirror image. This form is said to be *racemic*, taken from the Latin *racemus*, for a cluster of grapes.

When Pasteur announced the result of his experiment of separating the right and left handed mirror image crystals and dissolving them together, giving a solution with no display of light bending, **Jean Baptiste Biot** (1774-1862), a celebrated French physicist who had pioneered work with quartz crystals, asked Pasteur for a demonstration. Biot, after serving in the artillery in 1792 fighting the British, attended the École Polytechnique after which he was appointed professor of mathematics at the University of Beauvais. In 1800 he moved to the College of France where he was active in a number of scientific studies, some of which were adventurous and dangerous. In 1804 he ascended in a balloon with a scientist friend, **Gay-Lussac** (1778-1850) to heights of up to three miles to make instrumental observations and determined, for example, that there was no difference in terrestrial magnetism. Biot's most notable work was in polarized light. It had been discovered a century and a half earlier that two rays of light emitted from an Iceland spar differed in properties. In 1815, seven years before Pasteur was born, Biot showed that many organic substances could rotate polarized light to the right or left whether they were liquids or solids in solution. In 1835 he found that hydrolysis of sugar would cause it to change its optical rotation. That, and related work, led him to believe that optical rotation was due to an asymmetry in the molecules. Biot's work was the foundation of the science of polarimetry for which, in 1840 he was awarded the Rumford Medal of the Royal Society.[1]

Pasteur's recognition by such a highly regarded scientist was a boost to the young man's career. He was on his way to fame, eventually honored by the Rumford medal of the Royal Society and a member of the Legion of Honor. Ten years after his work on twisting of light by mirror image crystals he discovered something else about right and left handed crystals. A plant mold growing in a mixture of the two kinds of crystals, therefore optically inactive, fed on only one kind of crystal, leaving what was left optically active. It was the first evidence of what is now generally accepted, that living tissue invariably uses only one of the right or left handed molecules. This finding, which at the time seemed to be of only scientific interest, one hundred years later became a crucial feature in the development and use of pharmaceuticals (See chapter 19).

SOUR WINE

Recognition of Pasteur's work with crystals led to his being made a member of the Legion of Honor. The erstwhile student once graded "mediocre" in chemistry had become famous. Upon completion of work for his doctorate in 1848 he was appointed professor of chemistry at the University of Strassburg, and in 1854, still in his early thirties, he became dean of the faculty of science at the University of Lille in the north of France. It was his understanding that he was expected in his teaching and research to be attentive to the problems of the area in which vineyards and wine production were important industries.[2]

Shortly after arriving at Lille, an industrialist named **Bigo** approached Pasteur with a problem. Monsieur Bigo was in the business of producing alcohol by fermentation of beet juice and complained that the alcohol was often spoiled by contamination with something that he could not detect. Pasteur visited Bigo's distillery several times, took samples of fermenting juice back to his laboratory, examined them under the microscope, and followed them through the fermentation process. It was known that yeast was an important part of fermentation of juices. Pasteur saw the globular yeast cells under the microscope and he noticed something else. In addition to the globular cells there were smaller elongated cells, more of them in some samples than others. In contrast to the prevailing belief, including that of the famous German chemist **Justus von Liebig** (1803-1873), that fermentation was purely chemical and that any objects present were simply part of the process, it dawned on Pasteur that the cells he saw were, as he called them, "living ferments," or as we say, living organisms. The organisms in the ferment were not only different in size and shape, they were also different in their effect on the ferment. The solution to Bigo's problem was to find a way to get rid of the bad ones.

Pasteur temporarily turned his attention to the similar problem vintners had with wines turning "sour" as they aged, costing the vintners millions of francs in lost production of quality wines. Changes that reduced the quality of wine took various forms: Bordeaux wines "turned," Burgundy wines became "bitter," and Champagne became "ropy." There were also similar problems with beer. Pasteur experimented with samples of good and sour wine and concluded that the lactic acid in sour wine came from the presence of the small elongated cells. Heat had long been used to preserve food from spoiling, but boiling wine was unthinkable. In the 1860s, as a shot in the dark he experimented with treating wine at various reduced temperatures and found that gentle heating to 150 degrees F. would stop production of lactic acid without impairing quality of the wine. He explained to the vintners that while it was necessary to have the good yeast cells to produce alcohol, it was necessary to get rid of the (bad) cells that produce lactic acid. And to do that it was necessary to gently heat the wine before aging. The vintners were horrified at the idea of heating their precious wine. But they were desperate for a remedy. Pasteur treated samples of wine with heat along with samples of untreated wine, and asked the vintners to wait six months for the samples to age. None of the heat-treated samples went sour. Some of the untreated wine did. The treatment, called *pasteurization*, is now used also in preservation of milk and other products.[3, 4]

Pasteur concluded that Bigo's problem with good and bad alcohol from fermenting beet juice was similar to that in wine and beer, and that the remedy would be similar.

SICK SILKWORMS

In 1862 the lucrative silk producing enterprise in central and southern France was in trouble. A disease was killing the silkworms—insects that produce the silk. Without thriving cultures of the "worms" it wasn't long before the silk farmers were on the brink of ruin. Pasteur's old teacher, **Jean Baptiste Dumas**, who was from the silk growing area, asked him to head a commission appointed by the Ministry of Agriculture to study the problem. Pasteur protested that he knew nothing about silk production. "All the better," said Dumas.

Silk is made by caterpillars, that is, the larvae, of silkworm moths, *Bombyx mori*, which feed on mulberry leaves. The moth, which measures two inches or more with wings spread, lays 300 to 500 eggs from which the caterpillars emerge. They grow to a length of nearly three inches and up to an inch thick. When fully grown their salivary glands secrete a protein material which they extrude into a tough, silken fiber. It's the strongest of all natural fibers, having the tensile strength of steel. They use it to spin their cocoons, which are formed from a continuous thread of silk from 800 to 1,200 yards long. After molting (shedding their skins) four times and maturing into adults, the moths emerge by cutting their way through the silk cocoon. In silk farming the cocoons are treated with steam or dry heat to kill the moths before they can damage the silk.

Legend has it that silk was discovered in 2697 BC in the garden of Chinese Emperor **Huang-Ti** when he ordered his wife, Empress **Si-Ling-Shi** to find out what was damaging his mulberry trees. She not only spotted caterpillars voraciously eating the foliage, but when she picked up a cocoon that had fallen into water and removed the outer debris, the cocoon unwound into a long silken thread. It was not long before the fabulous value of silk became evident. The emperor ordered the discovery kept secret under penalty of death, and for 2,000 years the Chinese held a monopoly on the world market for silk, much of it transported by camelback over the caravan route to Damascus, which was the distribution point to markets in the Middle East and Europe.

The Byzantine **Emperor Justinian** (ruled AD 527-565) was unhappy with the exorbitant prices he and his luxury-loving subjects had to pay for silk garments, so in AD 555 he sent two monks to China as spies to pry out the secret. They returned with silkworm eggs and mulberry seeds hidden in cane sticks. It wasn't long before silk farming was adopted in several Middle East and European countries, as well as in other parts of the world including the United States, with France eventually being the top producer and Italy a close second.

In 1865 Pasteur took his microscope with him to the heart of the silkworm farming area in the mountainous region of Cévennes where he set up a makeshift laboratory. One of the first things Pasteur learned was that sericulture is a labor-intensive endeavor requiring meticulous care, immaculate cleanliness, and inspections at every step from eggs to spinning the fiber, tasks the Chinese were comfortable with but which may not have been compatible with the French temperament. Pasteur found that the silkworms were afflicted with two diseases, the most serious being caused by a protozoan parasite. Some diseases caused by protozoa are difficult to control as attested to by the high mortality from the human parasite, *Plasmodium* sp., that causes malaria. Pasteur persuaded the silk farmers that they must destroy all of their worm cultures, thoroughly clean the nurseries, and start over again with carefully selected disease-free eggs.

Five years after Pasteur started his investigation of the problem, silk farming was back in profitable operation and continued to thrive until disrupted by the two world wars. Women were unhappy with the scarcity of silk hosiery and the agonizing choice limited to course cotton stockings. But in the 1930s, chemists of E.I. du Pont de Nemours and Company, of Wilmington, Delaware, discovered Nylon, a remarkably versatile product, capable, among other things, of forming a fiber said to be stronger than any known natural fiber. Chemist **Wallace H. Carothers** had a leading role in its development. It came to be used in a wide variety of consumer and industrial products, and in 1938 was introduced to the market in Nylon hosiery, almost equal in sheer beauty to silk, and less expensive.

THE CROOKED NECK FLASK

Pasteur's microscopic observations of crystals and yeasts led his inquisitive mind to speculate about the origin of life. Greek philosophers had taken a stab at it. **Aristotle** (384-322 BC) believed that living things could and did arise spontaneously from inorganic matter without the need for preexisting life. His pupil, **Theophrastus** (372-287 BC) doubted it, and **Lucretius** (95-55 BC), a Roman philosopher ahead of his time, concluded that "the earth has ceased to create life." But the prevailing view for more than 2,000 years from Aristotle to Pasteur's time was the doctrine of "spontaneous generation" of life.

William Harvey (1578-1657), a famous English physician (see chapter 6), took some of his views almost straight out of the book of Aristotle. He had a theory that the unity of all life could be found in the egg, from which all creatures evolved. Harvey said, "All animals, even those that produce their young alive, including man himself, are evolved out of the egg." A contrary theory, called the theory of preformation, was held by **Jan Swammerdam** (1637-1680), a Dutch naturalist, who held that all animals evolve in the embryo from previously created parts. His theory was also contrary to the popular belief in the spontaneous generation of lower organisms. But the existence of spontaneous generation remained the more popular view. Pasteur was uncomfortable with the spontaneous generation idea because it conflicted with the teaching of his religious upbringing that all forms of life on earth were created in the beginning at the same time. His religious view also led him to reject **Charles Darwin's** (1809-1882) theory of the origin of species.

Pasteur's experiments with fermentation and control of yeast cells aroused an interest in showing that small organisms do not arise from dead matter. **Jean Baptiste Biot** (1774-1862), the French physicist, warned Pasteur that it would be a formidable and controversial problem to try to disprove the views and findings of respected scientists. **Jöns Jakob Berzelius** (1779-1848), an influential Swedish chemist, had believed in spontaneous generation, even though **Lazzaro Spallanzani** (1729-1799), an Italian biologist, ran experiments in 1768 that refuted the claims for spontaneous generation. He boiled for as long as three quarters of an hour solutions that would be expected to breed microorganisms, then sealed the flasks. No growth appeared. The results were influential in stimulating improvements in food handling. However, **Ernst Haeckel** (1834-1919), a German naturalist, and others, maintained that by heating the air above his solutions Spallanzani destroyed some vital principle that would otherwise cause organisms to appear spontaneously.

Pasteur finessed that objection. He and others had observed that when a nutrient broth was exposed to the air with its ever-present dust particles floating around, microorganisms would invariably develop, suggesting to some people the spontaneous origin of life. Pasteur, in 1860, boiled meat and left the extract exposed to air in a flask, but the flask had a long, narrow neck which he bent down, then up. Air could enter the tube but dust or other small particles would settle at the bend and could not contaminate the broth. No organisms developed in the broth. Pasteur had nailed it. He had demolished an erroneous idea that had been kicked around since the time of Aristotle, 2,100 years earlier, and still adhered to by scientists generally. Pasteur reported his results at a meeting at the Sorbonne on April 9, 1864. A committee of scientists who evaluated his experiments declared them valid. They led to a better understanding of the need for safe handling of food and contributed to the emerging science of bacteriology.

THE GERM THEORY

Louis Pasteur's microscopic studies on yeast cells, methods for protection of food, wine, or beer from spoiling, a way to prevent the disastrous disease of silk moths, all had led him to believe that diseases must be spread by germs too small to be seen except under a microscope. His so-called germ theory of disease has been described by **Isaac Asimov**, the science historian, as "…probably the greatest single medical discovery of all time, for only through an understanding of the nature of infectious disease and the manner of its communication could it be brought under control." The idea that diseases were caused by an unseen organism was contrary to the belief held for thousands of years that diseases were not communicable but were caused by the curse of spirits, or vapors, or one or more of a person's so-called humours being mysteriously out of balance.

Even before Pasteur began his investigations of yeast in wine and beer, and diseases of silkworms, **Friedrich Henle** (1809-1885), a German medical pathologist and anatomist, had speculated that diseases were caused by microorganisms, but he had no evidence to support the idea so his ruminations were dismissed. A Hungarian physician, **Ignaz Philipp Semmelweis** (1818-1865), was puzzled by the high frequency of childbed fever and its appalling death rate in Vienna hospitals, while women who gave birth to children at home with only the help of ignorant midwives more often survived. He reasoned that it was the doctors who were carrying the disease from the delivery rooms to women in labor they were treating. He ordered doctors under him to wash their hands in chemicals. Childbed fever declined drastically, but doctors did not take kindly to washing, which to them was simply a foolish annoyance. So when Hungary, which was under the domination and part of Austria, revolted in 1849 but lost in the attempt, the infuriated doctors used it as an excuse to force the annoying Hungarian out of the country. The result was a drastic increase in childbed fever. Semmelweis relocated to a hospital in Budapest where he again instituted his antiseptic procedure and virtually eliminated childbed fever there also. Unfortunately, he injured himself while treating a sick patient and came down with an infection that killed him before he could live to see antiseptic measures prevail under Pasteur, Lister, and others.

In general, the "germ theory" was seen as an outrageous idea that contradicted what had been believed since the time of Aristotle and Galen about the cause of diseases, which could be unfriendly spirits, the wrath of gods, or something mysteriously acquired from a miasma in the atmosphere. The upstart idea of germs was a theory too hard to swallow. But a brilliant German physician nailed it by proving the microbial causes of several diseases. (See The Explorer, chapter 8)

CHAPTER 8

THE EXPLORER

Robert Koch (1843-1910), a German physician-bacteriologist, twenty-one years junior to Pasteur, was a worthy rival in discovery and contributions to healing. His findings supported Pasteur's pioneering work and encouraged Pasteur in his classic work on immunization. Koch's work helped to remove any excuses for the blatantly unsanitary practices common among the elite doctors. Among his major accomplishments, Koch established microbiology on a sound scientific basis, using methods and innovations that have become standard practice even today.

Robert Koch was born in Hanover (later lower Saxony) as one of thirteen children of a mining official. He studied medicine at the University of Göttingen where he received his degree in 1866. At the time it seemed farfetched that he would become famous, for he dreamed of becoming an explorer. His wife wasn't understanding of his ambitions, so he divorced her and in shocking defiance of the social standard of the time married a younger woman more in harmony with his thinking. He settled down to ground-breaking explorations in science, medicine, and healing.

He served as an army surgeon in the Franco-Prussian war, then set up practice as a country doctor near Breslau. It was there that he became familiar with the devastating effects of anthrax on livestock. He obtained bacteria from the spleen of diseased cattle and was able to prove that they were the cause of anthrax. He discussed his work with **Ferdinand Julius Cohn** (1828-1898), a German botanist and bacteriologist who was teaching at the University of Breslau. Cohn was so impressed that he sponsored a paper written by Koch that led to his professional recognition.

Koch developed a scientific system for determining the causative agents of diseases that set a lasting pattern for the profession. His work with bacteria led him to establish guidelines for determining whether a particular microorganism is the cause of a disease. He said that the microorganism must be present in the diseased animal, and that after being cultured it must be capable of causing the disease in a healthy animal, and finally, the microorganism taken from that animal must be identical to those taken from the original animal. His guidelines continue to be the standard today for identifying causative agents of disease. For example he transferred the bacteria from anthrax diseased animals to mice and recovered the same bacteria again after transferring the infection from mouse to mouse. He also learned how to culture the bacteria outside the body by using blood serum kept at body temperature. Further, he was able to detect the formation of spores, a feature of anthrax that makes it a terribly dangerous disease, the spores being able to survive in the soil for many years.

Koch moved to pursue his studies in Berlin where he developed some important techniques, among them the use of aniline dyes for staining bacteria to make them easier to see under the microscope. An important innovation was the use of gels as an alternate to liquid nutrients. A gel such as agar-agar, derived from seaweed, is not a nutrient but serves as a base for nutrients. The semisolid gel keeps colonies of microorganisms separate instead of being swished around in a liquid media. An assistant, **Julius Richard Petri**, devised shallow glass dishes with protective glass covers in which to culture bacteria. The *Petri dish* is an indispensable item in microbiology labs today.

Koch went on to make landmark discoveries in pathogenic microorganisms. The one that would bring the most notoriety and fame was his discovery in 1882 of the bacillus, *Mycobacterium tuberculosis*, that causes tuberculosis, also known as consumption or the "white plague". It was a scourge in Europe during the Industrial Revolution when congestion and overcrowding in cities contributed to the spread of contagious diseases, especially those that were spread air-borne and by close contact, like tuberculosis. Koch tried to find a cure for it and announced in 1890 that he had discovered one, but was deeply disappointed to learn later that he was mistaken. While knowledge of the cause was crucial to prevention, it remained for the discovery and use of antibiotics to provide a cure of tuberculosis. (See Chapter 17.)

Koch investigated cholera and bubonic plague during a trip to Asia in 1883. Cholera, called "the scourge of the nineteenth century" had spread from Asia to other parts of the world in seven pandemic episodes. Beginning in 1817, it spread from Bengal to China, through Persia to Egypt, from Russia to England, by 1832 reaching North America, and to Latin America in the following year. Koch's discovery of the causative agent, the bacterium *Vibrio cholerae*, was immensely important in dispelling the belief in miasmas and the futile attempts to prevent the spread of the disease by building large fires to destroy the supposedly air-borne cause. And it was crucial knowledge for the only preventive measure—elimination of human feces from the water supply. For Koch's discovery of the cholera bacillus, he was given a government grant of the equivalent of $25,000 and was appointed professor of hygiene at the University of Berlin in 1885. The cure for cholera, now known to be the prompt replenishment of lost fluid, is simple and easily applied, but control is still impeded in parts of the world where the disease is endemic due to truly massive pollution of major water sources such as the Ganges River in India and Bangladesh.

Continuing his search for the causative agents of diseases, Koch's studies between 1896 and 1906 enabled him to make the monumental discovery that some diseases are not caused by pathogen infection directly but by transmission through carriers such as insects. He determined that the plague bacillus is transmitted to humans by fleas that live on rats, and that sleeping sickness is transferred by the bite of the tsetse fly. This information was crucial in leading investigators to discoveries of the ways in which other vector-borne diseases are spread such as malaria and yellow fever by certain species of mosquitoes.

Koch received the 1905 Nobel prize for medicine and physiology in honor primarily for his discovery of the cause of tuberculosis.

Alfred Bernhard Nobel (1833-1896), was a Swedish inventor. His father was a noted (self-educated) inventor who had become famous for inventing a submarine mine that was bought by the Russian government. The elder Nobel was hired to supervise its manufacture. In 1850 Alfred Nobel's father sent him to the United States where he spent four years studying under John Erickson, (1803-1889) a Swedish-American inventor who had become a U.S. citizen. When the young Nobel returned to Russia he found his father engaged in the study of explosives. At the time, there was an interest in nitroglycerin which had been discovered a decade earlier by Ascanio Sobrero (1812- 1888), an Italian chemist.

Young Nobel's stay in the United States gave him visions of a continent to be brought under control, He saw how roads could be blasted out of mountains, canals dug, and foundations laid without the weary muscles of countless human beings. While experimenting in a safe place Nobel made an accidental discovery. The nitroglycerin container had leaked saturating the packing material of diatomaceous earth which, however, seemed to remain perfectly dry. He found that the mixture could be handled safely and could not be set off without a detonating cap. He called the mixture "Dynamite." The myriad uses for the explosive power of dynamite made Nobel enormously wealthy. He was a bachelor, moody, lonely, and unpopular. He actually thought that his explosives would outlaw war by making it too horrible.

After he died, Nobel left his entire estate, $9,200,000, to establish annual prizes (the Nobel Prizes) in five fields: Peace, Literature, Physics, Chemistry, and Physiology and Medicine. In 1969, a sixth award in Economics was added but it is separately funded.

The prizes carried a cash award of about $100,000 but the money is not to be compared to the honor of the Nobel Prize. The first to honored with a Nobel Prize was Wilhelm Conrad Roentgen (1845-1923), a German physicist, for his discovery of X rays, X being the usual mathematical symbol for the unknown.

The Nobel Institute in Sweden is named for Alfred Nobel. And because element 102 was first isolated there in 1958 it was named Nobelium.

CHAPTER 9

THE IMMUNIZERS

Few advances in health and healing have done more to alleviate suffering and prolong healthful lives then the discovery of ways to immunize people against the onslaught of diseases. Faltering steps toward that end began against the scourge of smallpox, a terrible disease that had afflicted humanity since the beginning of recorded history. Some of the ancient so-called "plagues" were probably in reality epidemics of smallpox. The disease again flared up as the worst affliction during the late Middle Ages. The disease had gradually declined after the series of disasters during the last half of the 1300s. Although there were still sporadic outbreaks, it was no longer the frightful calamity it had been, probably because of the death of many of the more susceptible people and, maybe more importantly, that a high percentage of the surviving population may have developed immunity.

Smallpox, unlike many diseases that occur in both people and animals, or those that are transmitted from one person to another by animals, it is strictly an affliction of humans. It was often fatal, but even when the patient survived, it left the victim disfigured with ugly puckered *pockmarks*. It became evident that people who survived never had a second attack. However, the disease struck people with different degrees of severity, and even people with mild cases were just as protected from further attacks as those who survived severe cases. This knowledge led to the idea that if one could somehow acquire the disease from someone with a mild case of the illness, it would be better than taking a chance on catching the disease from someone with a severe or even fatal case.

In 1713, a prominent English poet, **Lady Mary Wortley Montagu** (1689-1762), whose husband was the British ambassador to Turkey, brought back the news that people in that country were being inoculated with pus from the sores of those who appeared to have mild cases of the disease. She had her son inoculated while the family was still in Turkey. But the practice was risky. Sometimes inoculation with pus from the pustules of a patient with a mild case would cause serious or even fatal illness. It was like playing Russian roulette. But fear of the disease was so great that many people submitted to inoculations, and the practice continued for more than three fourths of a century despite the added effect that it tended to further the spread of the disease. It was called *variolation* from *variola*, the medical term for smallpox. The danger that variolation would be a cause of serious disease, not a cure, probably kept it from becoming popular.

One of the greatest breakthroughs in medical science came in 1796 when an experiment was conducted by **Edward Jenner** (1749-1823), a country doctor who found another way to protect people from smallpox. Jenner, the son of a clergyman, lost both his father and mother at the age of five. After some schooling under the care of an older brother, he was apprenticed to a surgeon and eventually obtained a medical degree from St. Andrews. His practice among the country folk of Gloucestershire was not enough to fully absorb the fertile mind of this talented man whose interests ranged from music and poetry to natural history. He was sufficiently accomplished in the latter to be hired to prepare and organize the zoological specimens collected by Captain Cook on his first voyage to the pacific in 1768. He was offered the position of naturalist on Cook's second voyage but he decided to stay at home with his medical practice.

The time was one in which smallpox continued to be frightfully prevalent. Very few people escaped the disease, which displayed varying degrees of virulence. During the worst epidemics as many as a third of the patients died. But, as previously noted, people who survived were never known to have a second attack. The disease induced immunity.

Jenner had among his clients people who were in the dairy business. A common condition of dairy cattle was a disease called *cowpox* that was similar in some ways to smallpox but much milder. Cowpox appeared as pustules, small sores containing pus, on the legs of the animals. Some of the handlers, including milkmaids, who regularly came in close contact with the cows would get similar pustules, especially on their hands. Except for a local annoyance which lasted for a short time, they did not get sick and after one such incident they were immune to any future outbreak of the cowpox sores.

The fear of smallpox during the epidemic was so great that physicians were sometimes called upon to provide smallpox inoculation. Most of Jenner's clients refused in the belief that it would be useless. It was common knowledge, according to the dairy people, that anyone who had ever had cowpox would not get smallpox. The tradition was supported by the experience of those who submitted to inoculation. It never produced smallpox in anyone who previously had cowpox. The tradition that milkmaids who had acquired cowpox were immune to both cowpox and smallpox may explain why milkmaids are always depicted with a fair and attractive complexion.

The connection between cowpox and resistance to smallpox did not escape Jenner's attention. He thought that if he could transmit cowpox to a person who might be in danger of acquiring smallpox, they would be as safe from the ravages of that terrible disease as the milkmaids. But he knew that it would be hard to get the idea across to a profession notoriously cool to any practice that would deviate from the thousand year-old dictates of Galen. He decided to conduct a frighteningly bold experiment. On May 14, 1796, a milkmaid named **Sarah Nelmes** who had cowpox allowed Jenner to take fluid from a blister on her hand and inject it into an eight-year-old boy named **James Phipps** who, as expected, got cowpox. Jenner waited six weeks, then rubbed a scratch in the boy's arm with pus from a sore of a man who had smallpox. If the boy had died or become seriously sick Jenner would have been a criminal. But the boy had no ill effects. Jenner sent a description of his experiment to the Royal Society, but publication was refused. The members thought the boy's failure to acquire smallpox was mere happenstance. Jenner saw that the test would have to be repeated, but he had to wait two years to find another patient with active cowpox. The second experiment, in 1798, was equally successful, and Jenner felt free to publish his results. In 1798 he published a small book, *An Inquiry into the Causes and Effects of the Variole Vaccine*. The Latin word for cow is *vacca* and cowpox was called *vaccinia*, so Jenner coined the word *vaccination* to describe the procedure. He had founded the science of immunology.

The horrors of smallpox made a vaccination quickly and widely accepted. Jenner became an honored worldwide celebrity. Members of the British royal family were vaccinated. The British Parliament in an uncharacteristic move awarded Jenner 10,000 pounds in 1802 and another 20,000 pounds in 1806. Twelve thousand people were vaccinated in

England in eighteen months. A hundred thousand people were vaccinated the world over by 1800. In Germany Jenner's birthday was celebrated as a holiday, and Bavaria made vaccination compulsory. The Dowager Empress of Russia sent a ring to Jenner and had the first child in Russia to be vaccinated named **Vaccinoff** and educated at the expense of the nation.

Napoleon ordered all the men of his army vaccinated and struck a medal in Jenner's honor. Great Britain, after a short peace, had resumed its war with Napoleonic France during which some British civilians were held captive. They were released because Jenner's name was mentioned on a petition to Napoleon. The vaccine came to the New World on a ship from Spain that contained children who were vaccinated from the sores of those who had been previously vaccinated. The American Indians, never having been exposed, for at least the twelve thousand or so years of their existence in the New World, to the onslaught of European and Asian diseases brought by the Spanish explorers and later colonists, were lacking in immunity and resistance to the foreign diseases. They suffered grievously from smallpox. In appreciation of their deliverance from its horrors by vaccination, the Amerindians sent a deputation to England with gifts to thank Jenner personally.

The medical profession was in no hurry to honor Jenner. In 1813 he was proposed for membership in the College of Physicians but stipulated that the country doctor be tested in the classic methods of medicine, meaning the millennia-old moth-eaten theories of Galen. To Jenner's credit he refused, and was not elected.

For the first time in the experience of humanity a major disease had been conquered, and since then it has never been a problem in the medically advanced countries. But smallpox remained virtually uncontrolled in other parts of the world where as recently as 1966, millions of people contracted the disease and 2 million died every year.

Neither Jenner nor anyone else knew why vaccination worked and they had no idea how the method might be used to protect against other diseases. It was another half century before the puzzle of the cause of a disease was unraveled by a French chemist, **Louis Pasteur** (1822-1895), whose discoveries led to understanding the immunization principal, and how it could be used to control other diseases.

CHAPTER 10

PASTEUR'S VACCINATION

Pasteur had suffered a paralytic stroke in 1868 during his studies of the silkworm disease that left him severely handicapped. Yet, when France declared war on Prussia in 1870 out of fear that a Prussian alliance with a united Germany would upset the balance of power in Europe, Pasteur volunteered for service. He was politely turned down and told to stay with his microscopic study of diseases. But he got some patriotic satisfaction by returning an honorary medical degree that had been awarded by the Prussian University of Bonn.

France was overwhelmingly defeated in the following year but the war had lasted long enough for Pasteur to be shocked by what was happening to injured soldiers in the military hospitals. He resolved to persuade doctors to prevent infection by boiling their instruments and steaming their bandages. It took the courage of his convictions because he had no medical degree and no standing in the medical profession. But Pasteur's prestige forced them to accept his instructions. The results were so beneficial that in 1873 Pasteur was honored by being made a member of the French Academy of Medicine. Science historian **Isaac Asimov** opined, "…there was a growing suspicion (and a firm conviction nowadays) that he was the greatest physician of all time."

Pasteur's attention turned to anthrax, a dreadful disease of livestock with no known cure and no known way to prevent it. **Robert Koch** had discovered the bacterial cause of anthrax in 1876. Pasteur confirmed it and used cultures of it to prove conclusively the validity of the germ theory of disease. He found that a good culture media was urine in which he transferred the bacteria to fresh tubes of it 100 times without losing any of the bacteria's virulence. He carried knowledge of the disease a step further by finding that the germs were sometimes present as spores in the ground where they could be a danger to animals for many years. The immediate solution to Pasteur was to kill the diseased animals, burn their bodies, and bury them deep in the ground. But he was convinced that the real answer to the anthrax epidemic was to find a way to prevent it.

The English physician, **Edward Jenner,** had in 1798 found a way to prevent smallpox by injecting people with fluid from pustules of someone infected with cowpox, a much milder pox disease. Pasteur faced a dilemma. There was no mild form of anthrax. Infection by the bacteria that cause it was always fatal. He found a clue to the answer in his studies of bird cholera. While still working on the anthrax problem he studied cholera in chickens which were afflicted with an epidemic of the disease. He prepared cultures of the cholera bacteria in tubes of broth which he kept going by repeatedly transferring portions to fresh broth. Otherwise they would die out in their own waste similar to the way yeast cells die after converting sugar to their poisonous waste, alcohol, during fermentation of wine. In one experiment to inoculate chickens with the cholera disease, Pasteur took his sample from a culture that had gone longer than intended. The chickens became slightly sick but did not die, so he inoculated them again with bacteria from a fresh culture. To Pasteur's astonishment they remained healthy. He is reported to have exclaimed to his associates, "Don't you see that these animals have been *vaccinated*?"

Repeated experiments always gave the same results. Pasteur had developed for the first time immunization of a bacterial disease. In honor of Jenner, Pasteur continued to call the method **vaccination** even though there was no *vaccinia* (cowpox) disease involved. The discovery is a classic example of Pasteur's gift of serendipity, that is, a talent for observing and comprehending the meaning of unexpected results. The word, serendipity, was coined from Horace Walpole's tale *The Three Princes of Serendip* (Ceylon) who had a talent for making discoveries from chance observations. Serendipity is characteristic of many successful researchers.

Pasteur returned to his anthrax studies encouraged by the knowledge that it was possible to produce attenuated bacteria. This time instead of waiting for the culture to expire in its own waste, he killed the bacteria with heat and used the slurry of dead bacteria to inoculate sheep. The vaccination worked. After repeatedly and successfully immunizing sheep against anthrax, he announced the results. There was widespread skepticism and demands for a demonstration to which Pasteur gladly complied by conducting a controlled test using 25 vaccinated sheep and 25 untreated sheep and injecting all 50 sheep with anthrax bacteria. All of the unvaccinated sheep died. All of the vaccinated sheep remained healthy.

Despite the spectacular success with anthrax, Pasteur's greater acclaim was from his work on rabies, or hydrophobia. This time he was dealing with a disease of people, and one that was always fatal. There was no cure and no way to prevent it if the victim was bitten by a rabid animal. Pasteur undertook to find the causative germ, but could not find any. He was able to pass the disease from diseased animals to healthy ones and this led him to speculate that the germ must be too small to be seen under a microscope. In this he was correct but it would not be until nearly a half century later that his guess would be validated in 1935 by an American biochemist, **Wendell Meredith Stanley** (1904-1971). Working on the tobacco mosaic disease, he was able to isolate the causative agent. He believed that the agent must be a protein, so he crushed infected leaves and put the filtered juice through the established procedure for crystallizing proteins. He obtained clear crystals and found that they would cause the mosaic disease when dissolved and injected into healthy tobacco plants. He called the agent a *filterable virus*. "Virus" is Latin for poison. A crystalline substance, capable of being reproduced in the infected organism and perpetuating a disease seemed to be on the boundary between life and non-life. The finding stimulated a prolonged controversy, protagonists arguing that a virus must be either living or nonliving like a peace of flesh. Since Stanley's work many other viruses have been crystalized, and they have all turned out to contain nucleoproteins, similar in that respect to genes. The fact that viruses can reproduce themselves argues strongly in favor of the view that they are living. Stanley was awarded a share of the 1946 Nobel Prize in chemistry.

Pasteur, having determined that extracts from animals with rabies would cause the same disease when injected in healthy animals, found that he could culture the causative substance in nerve tissue, and proceeded to produce attenuated cultures of the invisible virus. He found that spinal cords taken from rabbits that had died of rabies and kept for two weeks in a dry, sterile condition produced extracts that were almost non-virulent in animals.[1] Would they be safe and effective in humans? When a nine-year old boy, **Joseph Meister**, who had been severely bitten by a rabid dog was brought to his attention, Pasteur was faced with a dilemma. His work on immunization had been in the role of preventing disease before infection, not curing it. But with rabies he saw a window of opportunity. Symptoms of rabies are slow to develop. Perhaps administration of an attenuated agent early in the incubation period would be beneficial. On July 7 1885, he injected the young boy with attenuated rabbit spinal cord, and followed with a total of twelve inoculations of progressively more potent virus up to virus that was fully potent in untreated spinal cord from an infected rabbit. The boy never showed symptoms of rabies and returned home in good health. He was honored later by being given the job of gatekeeper at the Pasteur institute in Paris. When the German invaders in 1940 ordered him to open Pasteur's burial crypt, instead of complying he committed suicide.[2]

The second rabies patient of Pasteur was a shepherd boy of fourteen, **Berger Gupille**, who had been bitten by a rabid dog while trying to protect some younger boys from attack. Pasteur's vaccine administered six days after the boy was bitten saved him also. A statue in the yard of the Pasteur Institute shows the shepherd boy struggling with the rabid dog.[3]

Subsequently, vaccines have been produced for many diseases, having prevented illnesses and saved millions of lives, especially crucial in immunizing children. Vaccines are available in the United States for the following diseases:[4]

Adenovirus (only for U.S. armed forces), anthrax, cervical cancer (papilloma virus), cholera, diphtheria, meningitis (Hermophilus influenzae, type b), hepatitis A, hepatitis B, influenza, Japanese encephalitis, measles, meningococcal meningitis, mumps, pertussis (whooping cough), plague, pneumococcal infection (meningitis, pneumonia), polio, rabies, rubella (German measles), tetanus, tuberculosis, typhoid, varicella (chicken pox), yellow fever.

Clearly, the legacy of Louis Pasteur and Robert Koch has had an enormous impact on the health and welfare of a large part of the world.

Different types of vaccines are used depending on the nature of the disease. For example, diphtheria and tetanus bacilli do their damage by producing toxins, so attenuated bacilli are not used. Instead, the vaccines consist of the toxic products of the bacilli. Two or more vaccines are sometimes administered at the same time or together. A series of inoculations in children beginning at age of two months consists of vaccines for diphtheria, tetanus, and pertussis in a combination referred to as DTP. Some people criticize the use of DTP in infants believing that an organic mercury compound used as a preservative may be one thing responsible for the surging increase in autism. Physicians contend that there is no evidence of harm from the mercury in DTP, but the extreme toxicity of organic mercury compounds would call for an intensive study to firmly establish the *lack of harm*, taking into consideration the well known fact that the effect of poisons follows in general a bell curve similar to what is sometimes called a "normal" curve in which some members of the population are seen as resistant to high doses while other individuals are harmed by extremely low doses.

Two types of polio vaccines were produced. The Salk vaccine, developed by **Jonas Edward Salk** (1914-1995), an American physician and microbiologist, consists of polio virus killed with formalin. It was introduced in a mass field trial in 1954, and released in the United States in 1955. During its early use there was some hastily prepared vaccine that caused 200 cases of polio and 11 deaths. Other than that accident, the Salk vaccine is seen as safe.

The other type of polio vaccine was developed by **Albert Bruce Sabin** (1906-1993), a Polish-American physician and microbiologist, who was the first to establish the growth of polio virus in human tissue outside the body. The Sabin vaccine consists of the three strains of attenuated polio virus. Sabin first tested it on himself, then on prisoner volunteers before it was introduced in 1957, but not used in the United States until 1960. It is popular because it can be taken by mouth instead of injection as required with the Salk vaccine. Rare cases of polio from the Sabin vaccine, especially in people with impaired immune systems, is always cause for concern.

Yellow fever is a dangerous virus disease transmitted by the bite of mosquitoes, primarily the backyard, barrel and water-hole type, *Aedes aegypti*. **Walter Reed** (1861-1902), an American military surgeon, led a research team that proved the mosquito transmission of yellow fever, and found in 1901 that the causative agent is a filterable virus. Before the mosquito-link was discovered epidemics swept through the southern United States and Cuba during the early 1900's, causing great suffering for many years. The epidemics were eliminated by vigorous control of the mosquitoes and protection of people exposed to them, but the disease remained endemic in portions of Central and South America, the Caribbean, and west coast of

Africa, areas where the "yellow jack" remained a threat to workers and military personnel as well as residents.

The yellow fever vaccine was developed by **Max Theiler** (1899-1972), a South African-American microbiologist. Theiler attended the University of Capetown but before finishing decided to pursue his studies in London. On arrival he was told that he would have to repeat his courses, so instead of complying he worked four years in a hospital where he gained practical experience. In 1922 he accepted a position at the Harvard University Medical School, then in 1930 moved to the Rockefeller Foundation in New York. Theiler found that he could infect monkeys with the virus, transmit the virus from monkeys to mice, from mouse to mouse, and back to monkeys, after which the virulence was diminished. He tested the vaccine on himself and colleagues, and it was used by the French in Africa during the 1930s and 1940s. In 1937 Theiler developed a second, safer vaccine by passing the virus through almost 200 chick embryos. It became the standard yellow fever vaccine in South America. Still without any academic degree, Theiler was awarded the 1951 Nobel Prize for medicine and physiology.

The most recent vaccine on the foregoing list is the Merck vaccine called Gardasil that is claimed to have been shown safe and effective against the two strains of human papilloma virus that most commonly cause cervical cancer. The virus is spread through sexual intercourse, and the key to the effectiveness of the vaccine is to administer it before exposure. A proposal to mandate that the vaccine be given to prepubescent girls stirred up a storm of criticism as an intrusion on parental guidance. Merck was reported to have launched an aggressive lobbying campaign for mandatory use of the vaccine, and even before reliability of the vaccine was fully established, at last 24 states from Virginia to California, introduced proposals to require Gardisil inoculations for middle schoolers. But attempts to legislate the proposals failed, so mandatory immunization of school children for papilloma virus never materialized.

In 2006 a vaccine for Herpes Zoster (Shingles) was also developed by Merck. Shingles, a reactivation of the chickenpox virus causes a painful rash which can persist for weeks to even years. The vaccine was originally developed for adults over 60 and is now recommended by the CDC for those over 50.

The crowning achievement in the use of vaccines was the eradication of smallpox. In 1966 the World Health Organization (WHO) decided to conduct a ten-year world-wide mass eradication program. A team of 50 full-time and 600 part-time workers was put under the direction of **Donald Henderson** (b.1928), an American physician. (Dr. **Frank Fenner** (1914-2010) was an advisor, appointed chairman in 1917.) They were eminently successful. The last officially recorded case of smallpox was in 1977 in Somalia. (The United Nations Food and Agriculture Organization (FAO) announced October 14, 2010, that a 16-year effort by FAO's Global Rinderpest Eradication Programme (GREP) had accomplished the goal of wiping out rinderpest, a disease of cattle caused by a virus similar to those that cause human measles and distemper in animals. Rinderpest has caused devastating losses in East Asia and Africa.) Samples of the smallpox virus were kept in two safe laboratories, one in Atlanta, USA and the other in Moscow. The last known fatality from smallpox was in 1978 when the virus escaped through the ventilation system of a laboratory in Birmingham. **Janet Parker**, a photographer working on an upper floor, caught the disease and died. All stocks of the virus other than the two samples kept for safe keeping in the United States and Russia were destroyed, but there is a nagging suspicion that samples may be secretly held by governments, or even independent groups such as terrorists, for potential use in biological warfare.

CHAPTER 11

OF PEAS AND PEOPLE

One of the greatest discoveries of all time, ultimately affecting health and well-being, was made by a man born into the impoverished life of an Austrian peasant.

Gregor Johann Mendel (1822-1884) was born in Heinzendorf, Silesia (now Hynčice in Czechoslovakia). The lord of the manor where his father was a peasant worker told Johann that his task was to tend the fruit trees, which was a fortunate assignment because it gave him early experience in horticulture. He desperately wanted an education, and with what support his parents could give, he helped by tutoring. After struggling to graduate from the gymnasium (equivalent to high school) and attending the Philosophical Institute for two years, he realized that his only chance for a higher education was to enter a nearby Augustine monastery that at the time was supporting the education of monks and priests to become teachers.

In 1843 Mendel entered the Abbey of St. Thomas in Brünn as a monk, at which time he assumed the name Gregor. (Brünn is now Brno in Czechoslovakia). He was ordained a priest in 1847, and in 1851 was sent to the University of Vienna where in a two-year stint, the maximum time the Abbey would give, he studied experimental physics, statistics, probability, atomic theory of chemistry, and other subjects. He failed his exams twice, maybe due as much to his professor's inability to comprehend the young man's flair for mathematics as to the experience of "exam nerves." Actually, he had a nervous breakdown. He was assigned part-time, without what we would call a "credential," to teaching the lower grades. His dilemma reminds one of Albert Einstein's high school physics teacher telling him that he would never amount to anything. However in 1854 Mendel became a science teacher at the Brünn Realschule.

At the monastery, while working a small plot of ground measuring 35 meters by 7 meters (about 115 feet by 23 feet) Mendel noticed that seedlings from pea plants often differed from their parent plants in strange mathematical patterns. To explain the puzzle, he embarked in 1856 on a series of sophisticated, scientifically rigid, replicated breeding experiments, along with probability calculations. He pollinated each plant by hand, covered all the flowers with bags to prevent unwanted pollination, and kept careful records.

Mendel found that some "charakters" of the pea plants disappeared in hybrid progeny and reappeared in later generations. For example, he crossed two strains of pea plants, one with smooth seeds and the other with wrinkled seeds. When the hybrid plants produced seeds they were all smooth. The wrinkled character had disappeared. Although invisible, whatever it was that caused the wrinkles had not been eradicated. For when he planted the smooth hybrids he found that they were not all the same. Three-fourths of the seeds the hybrid plants produced were smooth and one-fourth were wrinkled. Mendel called the smooth character *dominant*, and the wrinkled character *recessive*. He had similar results from crossing tall plants with dwarf plants, in which as it turned out, the tall character was dominant and the dwarf character was recessive. He meticulously worked out the mathematical ratios of plants from different crosses and showed conclusively that heredity was not by blending characteristics as Charles Darwin had assumed but by inheritance of distinct characteristics. Mendel postulated that the plants contained what he called "elements" that caused the dominant and recessive characters. Later, 44 years after Mendel first reported his findings, a Danish chemist-botanist, **Wilelm Ludwig Johannsen** (1857-1927) in 1909 proposed the word *gene*, from a Greek word meaning "to give birth to." This led to the all-inclusive word *genetics* and such words as *genotype*.

Mendel reported his findings in 1865 at a meeting of the Natural Science Society in Brünn. The uncomprehending members at the meeting were bored. No one asked questions, there was no discussion. He sent his paper at once to be published in the Transactions of the Brünn Natural History Society and submitted a second paper in 1869. Mendel had read Darwin's *Origin of Species*, published in 1859, but for some reason did not mention it in his papers even though his findings explained what Darwin had failed to fathom. Charles Darwin had not seen Mendel's papers nor heard of his work. So when he wrote *Variations of Animals and Plants Under Domestication* in 1868, he did not have the data on which to base a full explanation of inheritance. But a stab in the dark came remarkably close to inheritance, based on subsequently revealed facts. Darwin called it "pangenesis," in which every cell in the body had particles he called "gemmules" that were passed on to the next generation by eggs and sperm, resulting in the offspring having a blend of the parents characteristics. In this, he went astray, for one of Mendel's important findings was that the progeny are not a blend of the parents but instead inherit distinct characteristics.

Mendel thought that the lack of interest in his work might be due to others thinking of him as an amateur scientist. Hoping to get confirmation of the validity of his work, he submitted his papers to a prominent Swiss botanist, **Karl Wilhelm von Nägeli** (1817-1891) who could see no sense in Mendel's mathematical treatment of what he took to be purely a matter of botanical characteristics. He dismissed Mendel's paper with a contemptuous reply, although he offered to grow some plants from Mendel's seeds, but never did. In his major work, a book on evolution, he made no mention of Mendel. Nägeli's blundering was a tragically missed opportunity to advance the study of genetics by a generation.

Mendel communicated with other scientists about his work but it seems that none of them had the understanding to see the importance of a connection between mathematics and botany. After eight years of exploring the secrets of heredity on a small patch of monastery land, he ended his experiments in 1868 when the Abbot of the monastery retired and Mendel was appointed to replace him. The administrative duties plus his vanishing agility to bend and kneel in a pea patch cut that work short. He had worked diligently with thousands of plants on which he meticulously kept records on 12,835 of them. His publications in an obscure journal remained unread or, if read, uncomprehended. He died January 6, 1884, lonely and disheartened, never knowing that the Mendelian laws of inheritance would someday be acknowledged worldwide as the cornerstone of developments in the coming science of genetics.

We pick up the thread of the story of genetics a generation later when in 1886 a Dutch botanist, **Hugo Marie De Vries** (1848-1935) rediscovered Mendel's finding. De Vries earned an M.D. degree in 1870 and in 1878 became a professor of botany at the University of Amsterdam. He was deeply interested in Charles Darwin's thinking on evolution and puzzled over the gap in Darwin's work that lacked an explanation of how the changes in characteristics during evolution that Darwin described could occur. One day on a walk in the country he came across a field of American evening primroses, an introduced plant, and noticed that some of the plants were distinctly different from others. He took samples of the different kinds and grew them separately and in mixtures with results that were essentially the same as Mendel's.

De Vries was ready to publish his results in 1900, but on reviewing the literature first he was surprised to find that his finding had been worked out in detail by Mendel. Even more surprising, also in 1900, two other botanists, **Karl Franz Joseph Erich Correns** (1864-1933) a German, and **Eric Tschermak von Seysenegg** (1871-1962) an Austrian, unknown to De Vries and to each other had each worked out the laws of inheritance and had also found Mendel's paper. Although otherwise it would have meant great fame, all three admirably demonstrated the highest level of scientific integrity by acknowledging Mendel's priority. The rules of reproduction are still called the Mendelian Laws of inheritance.

Aside from De Vries' experiments, publications, and role in publicly removing the wraps from Mendel's work, he made a serendipitous discovery strictly his own that was directly related to filling the gap in Darwin's views. During his walks in the field, he noticed that occasionally a plant distinctly different from the others would appear, and by experimenting found that it would breed true in subsequent generations. It was a new principle of evolution by sudden change or *mutation*, a Latin word meaning "to change." More than just helping to explain inheritance as well as evolution, knowledge of mutations is crucial to dealing with disease microorganisms.

The year 1900 marked the beginning of more than a century of astounding discoveries and developments in genetics. Mendelian laws were found to apply broadly to all plant and animal life. Further work by scientists beyond Mendel's fundamental findings in a pea patch and De Vries discovery of mutations in a field of primroses galvanized a surge of productive work in genetics and heredity, eventually leading to improvements in nutrition and health, one of which is the most exciting possibility of healing so far in this century: the use of stem cells.[1]

PART III
BATTLE AGAINST INSECTS

12 INSECTS AND DISEASES

13 BAD AIR

14 YELLOW JACK

15 LOUSY WAR

16 PLAGUES AND *THE PLAGUE*

CHAPTER 12

INSECTS AND DISEASES

Insects—animals whose adult forms typically have six legs and one or two pairs of wings, or none, are more numerous than all other animals on earth. They've dominated the world for millions of years. They looked dinosaurs in the eye and ruled the sky before birds existed. They were, and are, both beauty and beast, our best friends and our worst enemies. They make honey and pollinate many kinds of plants that provide food in quantities and variety without which our diet would be bland and less nutritious. But insects live in a world of conflict. Some species eat others of their six-leg ilk. Some turn on humans as their prey, and the thirst for blood of these vampires causes great suffering—not from loss of blood but from the germs and parasites they carry.

The role of blood-sucking insects as vectors of diseases was unknown until study and experiments by doctors, scientists, and other investigators revealed the part they play and ways to bring them—and some of the diseases they carry—under control. But the game is not over. Complete control of insect-borne diseases that have killed millions of people every year since earliest historic times, continues to be a humanitarian goal.

IMPORTANT DISEASES CARRIED BY BLOOD-SUCKING INSECTS

Malaria causes at least a million human deaths each year. The disease is caused by a single-cell *Plasmodium* parasite transmitted by the bite of female *Anopheles* mosquitoes (male mosquitoes do not bite).

Yellow fever killed millions of people each year before the cause was discovered that led to a method of control. The disease is caused by a virus that is transmitted by female *Aedes* mosquitoes. Still a threat.

Typhus, once widespread, is still a danger. The disease is caused by rickettsia (similar to bacteria) that is transmitted by the body louse.

The plague, bubonic and related forms, are caused by a bacillus that is carried by rat fleas. Throughout the middle ages, before the cause of disease and its vector were known, epidemics raged repeatedly across Europe, wiping out up to three-fourths of the population in some areas.

Dengue fever, also called breakbone fever due to the severity of symptoms, affects close to 100 million people each year. The disease, caused by a virus, is transmitted primarily by *Aedes aegypti* mosquitoes. There is no specific vaccine or drug for dengue and control is complicated by the fact that *A. aeygypti* is a species that is active during the day. However, a vaccine has been developed that is said to be effective against three of the four strains of dengue. Also, experiments are underway to alter the genetics of the mosquitoes to limit their ability to reproduce.

Sleeping sickness, also called African trypanosomiasis, is caused by a protozoan parasite of the genus *Trypanosoma* which is transmitted by tsetse flies, of which there are several species. The principal vector in west and central Africa is *Glossina palpalis*. The disease kills people, cattle, horses and other animals in Africa. The so-called "tsetse area," a vast expanse of sub-Sahara forest, is virtually off-limits for safe or profitable activity.

Chagas disease, also called American trypanosomiasis, is caused by a *Trypanosoma* parasite that is transmitted by the inch long cone nose, kissing or assassin bug, *Triatoma Sp*. At least 10 million people in Central and South America are infected. The assassin bug spends the day in the ceiling, drops down at night and painlessly sucks blood until it is bloated and leaves a very painful, itching bite. Charles Darwin (1809-1882) described how during his explorations in Argentina, "I experienced an attack (for it deserves no lesser name) by the Benchuca, the great black bug of the Pampus." When Darwin returned to England he suffered a panoply of incapacitating symptoms including flatulence, palpitations, insomnia, and hysterical crying. Several people speculated that he may have been afflicted with Chagas disease.

Elephantiasis (Lymphatic filariasis) is caused by threadlike parasitic roundworms (filariae), of which there are three types; the most common is *Wuchereria bancrofti*. The worms grow and reproduce in the body where they can cause damage for many years. The word *elephantiasis* derives from the gross deformaties such as massive enlargement of the legs, breasts, and genitals. The disease may also cause damage to the kidneys and the lymphatic system. The filariae are transmitted by several species of mosquitoes. In 1877, Sir Patrick Manson (1844-1922), a Scottish physician working in Amoy, China, was honored for being the first person to determine that a disease could be transmitted by an insect. Lympatic filariasis still affects millions of people and is a major cause of life-long disability in Africa, Asia, Latin America, and the Pacific Islands.

West Nile virus, carried by mosquitoes from infected birds, recently appeared in the western hemisphere. Classified as an arbovirus, it is capable of causing febrile illness (West Nile fever) and may include headache, myalgias or gastrointestinal symptoms. According to the Centers for Disease Control and Prevention (CDC), sixty-two cases appeared in New York state in 1999 causing seven deaths. In 2012, there were a total of 5,674 cases causing 286 deaths throughout the US.

"River blindness", also known as Onchocerciasis, so-called from a small parasitic worm *Onchocerca volvulus* that is transmitted by the female blackfly, genus *Simulium*, that breeds in fast-moving streams. The blackfly, also called no-see-um, is a blood-sucking gnat, no larger than 1.5 to 2 mm long. No-see-ums bite during the day and are incredibly vicious biters. Agonizing itching, reduced vision, eventually blindness and other serious effects of the disease caused residents of affected areas, especially of western and central Africa, to move away from infested rivers to less fertile dry areas.

In the following chapters we will examine the human suffering from four of the above insect-borne diseases and the heroic accomplishments of scientists to bring them under control.

CHAPTER 13

BAD AIR

Malaria, carried by mosquitoes, is an ancient affliction. The disease is described in the writings of Hippocrates. An Italian named **Torti** is said to have named it "malaria" in 1753 because people believed it was caused by the bad air, *mal aria*, arising from swamps and marshes.

Malaria typically goes through repeated cycles of three stages: a chill in which the skin becomes pale and has the appearance of "gooseflesh, accompanied by more or less violent shivering during which the patient's teeth may chatter. Next is fever, the temperature rising during the chill. And third, there is general perspiration. The entire paroxysm may last a few hours, and may reoccur for years if not successfully treated.

It was not until 1880 that the cause was discovered by a French army surgeon, **Charles-Louis-Alphonse Laveran** (1845-1922) who, after examining blood from malaria patients found a parasite in the red blood cells. To everyone's surprise it was not a germ but a single-cell animal, a protozoon given the genus name *Plasmodium*. It was the first pathogenic microorganism discovered that was not a bacterium. Laveran was awarded the Nobel Prize in physiology and medicine in 1907.

A theory said to be held for many years by Italian and Tyrolese peasants was that it was mosquitos that carried the disease from person to person. In 1883, **A.F.A. King** published a paper that presented the idea of a mosquito-malaria relationship. And in 1897 **Ronald Ross** (1857-1932), a British physician, after collecting, feeding, and dissecting mosquitos, saw the parasite that had been detected by Laveran in human blood cells.

Ross was born in Almora, India. His father was a general in the British army who sent his son at the age of eight to England for his education. Ronald took up the study of medicine in which he was an indifferent student, preferring to dabble in writing poetry and music. But he received his medical degree in 1879 at the age of 22 after which he entered service in the British army in India where he was assigned to service at several command posts. In England he had met and became friendly with **Sir Patrick Manson** (1844-1922), a physician who had also served in the Far East where he founded a school in Hong Kong, that eventually became the University of Hong Kong. His work in the Far East led him to establish tropical medicine as a specialty, and when he returned to England he founded the renowned London School of Tropical Medicine in 1889. Manson is sometimes called the father of tropical medicine. He was knighted in 1903.

Manson told Ross that mosquitoes might be the agents for transmitting the malaria parasite discovered by Laveran. He suggested that mosquitoes could suck up the malaria parasites in human blood, then were crushed in food or water and ingested by people. Whenever Ross had the opportunity to do so he engaged in microscopic dissection of mosquitoes looking for Laveran's parasites. He found them but was not able to determine how they got into the human blood stream. He came close. He set up some experiments with sparrows (birds get bird malaria) in which he demonstrated that the parasites were transmitted from bird to bird by mosquitoes. That did not prove that the same thing was happening in humans, but it was strong circumstantial evidence that was widely accepted as the explanation for the method of transmission of human malaria. Ronald Ross was awarded the Nobel Prize in physiology and medicine in 1902 and was knighted in 1911.

But it remained for an Italian scientist to unravel the rest of the puzzle of the transmission of malaria from person to person. **Giovanni Battista Grassi** (1854-1923) got his medical training at Pavia but did not become a practicing physician. Instead, he devoted his career to zoology and parasitology. He and his co-workers, **A. Bignami** and **G. Bastianelli**, demonstrated that the malaria parasitic plasmodium is transmitted from human to human by the bite of the female mosquito, and further, that it was a particular kind of mosquito belonging to the genus *Anopheles*. They issued a preliminary report in 1898 and a more thorough one in 1899.

There was animosity between Ross and Grassi, each claiming priority and credit for the discovery of what they believed would wipe out the curse of malaria from the face of the earth. But it was the Britisher who was awarded the Nobel Prize and was knighted, leaving his Italian rival unrewarded.

Even after Ross's discovery there was still some skepticism about the mosquito's role. Patrick Manson, who was a believer, suggested in 1900 that a mosquito-proof hut be built in the Roman Campagna. Two investigators, **L. W. Sambon**, an entomologist and **G. Low**, built and lived in the building during most of the malaria season, taking the precaution of retiring inside after sunset, the favorite mosquito feeding time. They were successful in avoiding malaria. They sent malaria infected mosquitoes to London where **P. Thurburn Manson**, physician son of Patrick, and **George Warren** let themselves be bitten by the mosquitos with the result that they both developed malarial fever and had several relapses.[1]

That nailed it. The disease is spread by the injection of saliva from the bite of female mosquitos of the genus *Anopheles* (male mosquitos do not bite). The way was now clear to find a way to prevent malaria by attacking the mosquitos that carry the malaria parasite. Further studies showed that malaria is caused by several species of *Plasmodium* that cause different forms and severity of malaria. Different types of *Plasmodium* differ in the nature and severity of their attack, actually causing what are virtually distinguishable diseases. Also, various species of *Anopheles* carry the parasites, and they vary in their habits and abundance in different geographic areas. **William B. Herms**, an entomologist at the University of California, said, "... of the nearly 170 species of Anopheles only 26 are considered to be important vectors of malaria," citing a 1931 report of a survey made in India by **Major G. Covell**. Anopheles mosquitoes are especially abundant in the tropics, but are also prevalent in temperate areas.

Before ways were found to control mosquitos, malaria was a world-wide affliction. For example, in 1935 there were 900,000 cases of malaria in the United States even though by then the incidence in the country was declining. It is now under control in most temperate parts of the world but remains endemic, that is, perpetually epidemic, in tropical areas were it kills at least one to three million people a year, especially affecting young children. Although the disease is most prevalent in Africa, it continues to be near the number one of human diseases world-wide, rivaling HIV/AIDS in death rate, and causing untold misery in sickness, lowered vitality, and economic distress.

Mosquito abatement as the primary way to control malaria was pioneered by **L. O. Howard** who was chief of the United States Bureau of Entomology from 1894 to 1927. He described experiments he conducted in 1892 with oils sprayed on the surface of water in which mosquitoes were breeding.[2] Subsequent work over the years has confirmed that malaria is best prevented by controlling the aquatic larvae and pupae of *Anopheles*, accomplished by draining problem bodies of water, or by spraying the water with oil or insecticides. Neither draining nor spraying are always feasible in tropical areas where it is more practicable to kill the adult mosquitoes with insecticidal fogs, or by protecting against mosquito bites with screens and nets, and by applying repellents to the skin. In most temperate parts of the world malaria was brought under control primarily by drainage of mosquito breeding areas and the use of a spray, often by aircraft, of petroleum oil to form a film on the water that will kill the mosquito larvae and pupae. Insecticides other then oil were often not needed. Control of malaria in tropical areas is more difficult. With the discovery of the insecticidal properties of DDT (*dichloro-diphenyl-trichloroethane*) in 1939 by a Swiss chemist, **Paul Hermann Müller** (1899-1965), in a search for an organic chemical that might be poisonous to insects but harmless to most other forms of life, it finally became possible to bring malaria under control in large areas.

DDT came as a panacea to people in areas where the cost of effective mosquito control by the usual methods was prohibitive. Even the cost of medicines were, and still are, out of reach for many people. DDT was cheap and easy to apply to houses with little health hazard to the occupants and virtually no risk of environmental damage. By the 1970s, malaria was reduced from an estimated 2½-3 million people a year to where it was almost under control. Millions of lives were saved, and alleviating the debilitating effects of malaria improved the standard of living. Even the development of resistance did not make DDT completely ineffective, and besides, the chemical appeared to have some repellent effect.

But events elsewhere seemed to conspire against reducing tropical malaria to insignificance. Enthusiasm for the spectacular new insecticide, less costly and safer to use than anything heretofore known, resulted in it being used carelessly and excessively in controlling pests of plants. The first indication of trouble was that the wide spectrum of activity of the magic bullet against a large number of species caused it to be lethal against some species of beneficial insects. Infestations of pests not controllable with DDT, such as mites, were made worse. Next was the appearance of resistance, a result comparable to the development of resistance of microbes to antibiotic medicines, also largely the result of excessive and injudicious use of those wonder drugs. Worst of all, DDT is so stable that it persists almost interminably and builds up in the environment. It was found to be stored in the fat and to build up to high levels in animals high in the food chain, referred to as "biological magnification." Accumulation of high levels of the chemical in sea birds disrupted their physiology in a way that caused their egg shells to be too thin and weak for the young to develop and hatch normally.

Even before most of these adverse effects were discovered, there was strong opposition to the use of DDT. Anxiety was aroused when government agencies used the chemical in a long-standing effort to control (and futilely hoping to eradicate) the gypsy moth, *Porthetria dispar*, an insect imported to the United States from Europe in about 1869 by a scientist who hoped to cross it with silkworm moths to produce a hybrid that would be resistant to the silkworm disease. Some of the Gypsy moths escaped into the wild and soon were causing extensive damage to woodland, shade trees, and fruit trees in the northeastern United States. The larvae strip the foliage of both evergreen and deciduous trees, often killing them. Several eradication campaigns were conducted in 1956-1959. The original weapon against the caterpillars was poisonous lead arsenate, which was replaced by DDT dissolved in diesel fuel or kerosene and sprayed by aircraft, indiscriminately covering towns and dwelling areas as well as woodland. The effort aroused a storm of protest against DDT. People's noses had no way of distinguishing between the smelly solvents and the odorless DDT, nor could they believe that the irritating spray was safer than the discarded lead arsenate.

The most influential person in opposition to the use of DDT was **Rachel Louise Carson** (1907-1964), a biologist who became prominent for her writings on natural history and the environment. Carson graduated from Pennsylvania College for Women, received an M.A. from Johns Hopkins University and did postgraduate work at Woods Hole Marine Biology Laboratory. She had a long career with the U.S. Bureau of Fisheries, followed by the U.S. Fish and Wildlife Service where she was editor in chief of its publications.

Carson was a gifted writer. Her 1951 book, *The Sea Around Us*, won the National Book Award, and her 1962 book, *Silent Spring*, aroused an awareness of the danger of environmental pollution. Her main target was DDT, having experienced the massive spraying with DDT against the Gypsy moth. She wrote passionately, "No birds sang in the poison rain." She was convinced that DDT was harmful to both wildlife and people. Before she succumbed to cancer within two years of the publication of the best seller, it was said that she blamed it on DDT. *Silent Spring* became the virtual Bible for environmentalism, and it helped stimulate an enormous amount of research on pesticides. Research on DDT alone, good and bad, was probably more than any other chemical in history. The result was an unstoppable trend toward a ban on DDT.

In the United States the peak production of DDT was in 1959 when 156,741,000 pounds were manufactured, of which 78,682,000 pounds were used within the country. The amount used in the United States decreased steadily during the 1960s. By 1969 it was less than half that of a decade earlier, and continued to decline in the 1970s. Arizona had placed a moratorium on the agricultural use of DDT in 1969, and other states followed. West Germany placed a ban on DDT except for forest use in 1971. Sweden, Norway, and Denmark had already banned DDT. And finally, the U.S. Environmental Protection Agency announced a ban on DDT for almost all uses, effective December 31, 1972.

DDT continued to be used in other countries, most of it being supplied by a Los Angeles manufacturer, Montrose Chemical Company, which eventually was persuaded to stop production after being cited by outraged authorities for careless handling of the product. Equipment in the factory was inadequate for dust suppression, and sweepings from spillage had been routinely hosed down the sewer, vast quantities ending up in the ocean and sand and muddy bottom of Santa Monica Bay.

Other chemical companies were reluctant to supply what they perceived as a declining demand, and fear of law suits. People involved in malaria control were compelled to switch to pesticides that were more dangerous, more expensive, and less effective. Microbiologists **Abigail Salyers** and **Dixie Witt**, declared in their 2005 book, *Revenge of the Microbes*, "The consequence of this today is that the malaria rate, mostly among children, is back up to where it was before DDT spraying."[3]

The first medicine for treating malaria was the bark of the cinchona tree, first used by the Incas. Knowledge of it reached Europe in 1642. The active ingredient came to be known as quinine, a bitter alkaloid. It was the only treatment known for three centuries, but without it Europeans probably would not have been able to support their aggressive exploitation of tropical areas of the world. Eventually there was concern that because the only source of quinine was from a South American tropical tree the supply might be cut off during wars. The first substitute to be developed was a drug called quinicrine, also called Atabrin, developed and first used in Germany. It became the established drug for malaria when, in fact, quinine became unavailable during World War II.

Nowadays, relying on medicines to control tropical malaria is more than simply handing the patient a bottle of pills. In most cases, a blood sample should be examined to determine the presence of the parasite and the species of *Plasmodium* involved. The mature form of *P. falciparum*, the most dangerous type, may stay in the blood stream for months, and the mature form of *P. malariae* may persist in the blood stream for years, causing repeated attacks of malaria. The most commonly used drugs are chloroquine, quinacrine (Atabrin), and primaquine. The *Plasmodium* in *falciparum* areas has developed resistance, especially to the favorite, chloroquine. In that case the patient may take the traditional quinine or be given quinidine intravenously. Resistance is less common in other types of malaria, in which case the usual treatment is chloroquine followed by primaquine.

Research on the long-sought malaria vaccine, while promising, has not been successful. The most powerful, economically practical, weapons for control of tropical malaria remain the low-tech procedures: window and door screens, netting impregnated with an effective, long lasting, insecticide, and spraying the interiors of dwellings and outlying buildings.

When philanthropists **Bill Gates** and **Melinda Gates** conducted what they called a "Malaria Forum" in their home town of Seattle on October 16-18, 2007, they announced a sweeping plan challenging the world to eradicate malaria from the face of the earth. The scientists in attendance were stunned. Eradication had been tried in the 1960s with an ignominious defeat when the DDT rug was pulled from under the campaign. Smallpox is the only human disease that has been eradicated except for cultures of the pathogen in some highly protected labs. Smallpox and malaria, however, have one thing in common. Neither one has an animal reservoir that would have to be eradicated. But the nature and pathway of the malaria parasite is much more complex. In a statement after his speech, Bill Gates said he thought of eradication as a long-term proposition. "Multiple decades," he told reporters. Some thought it was a good idea to revive the lofty goal. Others thought a better plan would be to eliminate as many *pockets* of the disease as possible, attacking the most obvious targets first. As put by **Richard Feachem**, head of the Global Health Group: start by picking the "low hanging fruit."[4]

William Henry Gates III was born October 28, 1955 in Seattle. He wrote his first software program at the age of 13. While a sophomore at Harvard in 1975, he and his boyhood friend, **Paul Allen**, developed software for the first microcomputer. Gates was too bright for college. In his junior year he quit Harvard and, with Allen, founded Microsoft Corporation. His goal was to "put a computer on every desk in every home". He negotiated an exclusive license for an operating system called MS-DOS with International Business Machines (IBM), then the predominant manufacturer of personal computers (PCs). That, and the introduction of the Windows operating system, led to Microsoft becoming the world's most valuable technology company. There are now more than 1 billion PCs worldwide. As early as 1986, Gates was a paper billionaire, and in time became the world's richest man. His personal fortune is estimated by Forbes Magazine at about $58 billion. In June 2008, Gates announced his retirement, while remaining as chairman of Microsoft and giving attention to special projects. His time, energy and financial support would be devoted to projects in the developing world such as vaccines and related health benefits.[5]

Another philanthropist decided to join Gates in his crusade against malaria and related health problems. Warren Buffett, one of the world's three richest men, is chairman of Berkshire Hathaway, an Omaha company listed on the New York Stock Exchange at a price per share that is out of reach for most investors. He announced in 2007 that the bulk of his fortune would be managed for charitable purposes through the **Bill and Melinda Gates Foundation**, the world's largest private charity.

Warren Edward Buffett was born August 30, 1930, in Omaha, Nebraska. He attended Woodrow Wilson High School in Washington, D.C. after his father was elected a congressman in 1942. He attended the

Wharton School of Business at the University of Pennsylvania, then went to the Lincoln School of Business Administration at the University of Nebraska where he took his B.S. degree in 1950. He was not satisfied with the training he had received, so applied to the Harvard Business School and took the train to Chicago to be interviewed by a Harvard alumnus. Buffett said, "...all the Harvard representative saw was a scrawny 19-year-old who looked 16 and had the social poise of a 12-year-old....The interview lasted about 10 minutes and they threw me back in the water." So Buffett applied to the Columbia Business School and was promptly accepted. There he admired and respected the teaching of **Benjamin Graham,** author of *The Intelligent Investor*. Buffett received his M.S. in business administration in 1951. In 1965 he took majority control of Berkshire Hathaway, a textile manufacturer.[6]

Some of the pooled assets of Buffett's and Gates' billions can be expected to go toward the malaria project already launched by the Bill and Melinda Gates Foundation. They, and other good people who are battling malaria with their careers, expertise, experience, time, or money, are faced with moral as well as scientific and financial decisions. How does anyone appraise the value of one life in the millions of lives that might be saved by the use of a chemical having the low cost, safety, effectiveness, and low environmental damage from DDT (as used in malaria control)? Malaria fighters are especially concerned about the welfare of children. Carcinogenic effects, organ damage, and endocrine disruption at effective exposure levels of DDT are conceivable, but proof is thin and largely speculative. Virtually all of the thousands of chemicals used as medicines are admittedly poisons, their toxic effects euphemistically called "side effects." The FDA, medical profession, and patients accept side effects as part of the price of health, or of lives. That might be true of DDT in malaria control, or of a comparable material, if it exists. Side effects might be insignificant compared to the benefits.

In September of 2008, at the UN headquarters in New York City there was a meeting of high level personalities geared to the launch of a massive attack on malaria. They included Bill Gates and British Prime Minister Gordon Brown. The Global Malaria Action Plan (GMAP) came from the input of more than 250 people knowledgeable of the problem. It came from the work of Roll Back Malaria (RBM), a group of international agencies, public and private donors, and affected countries. The goal is to reduce malaria deaths to zero by 2015. The plan harks back to a vow in the 1950s to eradicate malaria that seemed to be on the verge of success but ended in humiliating failure after the banishment of DDT.

Researcher Christian Lengeler of the Swiss Tropical Institute was quoted as saying that the goal of zero deaths by 2015 is "totally unrealistic." But RBM is plunging ahead. The plan is to greatly promote the use of bed nets and indoor insecticide spraying. And pharmaceutical companies are still interested in developing a malaria vaccine. Private donations along with funding by governments and international organizations came to $1.1 billion in 2008. Bill Gates pledged $168 million for research on malaria vaccines. Progress is in the cards although the goal and its timing are in doubt.[7]

CHAPTER 14

YELLOWJACK

Yellow fever caused devastating epidemics during the late 1700s and throughout the 1800s in the warm areas of North and South America. *Yellowjack* refers to the yellow jack (flag) flown by ships signaling the presence of yellow fever aboard. They often came from a Caribbean island, usually Jamaica. A shout of "yellowjack" conveyed the warning in one word that a ship was coming in with the dreaded disease.

Yellow fever is an agonizing ailment that causes fever, bleeding, jaundice (yellow discoloration of the eyes and skin due to liver damage), and often black vomit from bleeding in the stomach. The disease is caused by a virus that is transmitted from person to person by the bite of a female mosquito, *Aedes egypti*. Before this was known, people either panicked and fled or tried all sorts of things as preventives. Burning tar, night and day, produced a suffocating atmosphere as a barrier to the supposed deadly miasma. Medical treatment usually involved purgatives, blood letting, and disinfectants in liberal amounts of which vinegar and especially carbolic acid were favorites. These days, people planning to visit endemic areas are advised to get an injection of yellow fever vaccine. There is a remote risk of serious side effects, but not as risky as being bitten by an infective *Aedes egypti*. The first vaccine for yellow fever was developed in 1930 by **Max Theiler** (1899-1972), a South African-American neurobiologist. (See Chapter 10).

Yellow fever struck Philadelphia in 1793 and returned in less severe epidemics several times up to 1800. It hit New Orleans in 1822 and returned nearly every year for the next 25 years. A flare up in 1847 took 2,306 lives. The epidemic of 1878 in Mississippi and surrounding states may have been the worst epidemic in North American history. By the middle of the nineteenth century the epidemic subsided in its northern range but increased in severity in the South. During a later flare up, there were more than 500 deaths a week although many people who were able to get away had fled. The epidemic struck Natchez, a city on the bank of the Mississippi River (later the site of a bloody civil war battle). A more pleasant memory of Natchez is the Trace Parkway, a beautiful drive that parallels a historic mail and migratory route along an old Indian trail running for 500 miles from Nashville to Natchez.

Aedes egypti is the most domestic of mosquitos. It fits comfortably in human habitations, finding it convenient to breed in rain barrels, discarded tires, pots and pans, or anything that will hold water long enough for their eggs to hatch, the larvae (wrigglers) to grow, the pupae to mature, and the adults to emerge. In warm conditions it hardly ever takes more than a week. Human blood meals are nearby. The bite is facilitated by the injection of a small amount of saliva containing an anti coagulant along with a lethal virus or whatever pathogen the insect might have picked up during a previous blood meal.

American forces of the Spanish American war lost 968 soldiers in combat, but 25,000 were reported to have died of yellow fever. The Spanish governor of Cuba appointed **Carlos Juan Finley** (1833-1915) to the Yellow Fever Commission to collaborate with the United States National Health Board in an effort to find out how the disease was acquired. Finley's father was a Scot who had emigrated to the West Indies where he became a physician. His son, Carlos Juan, obtained his medical degree in 1855 at Jefferson Medical College in Philadelphia. He gave a talk in 1881 at the Academy of Sciences in Havana in which he put forward the opinion that yellow fever was transmitted from person to person by mosquitos, although he said that he had no scientific proof of it. His colleagues called him "a crazy old man." Finley probably knew about the work of **Patrick Manson** (1844-1922), a Scottish physician, who found by experiments that mosquitos transmit a worm, the filaria parasite, that causes filariasis, otherwise known as elephantiasis. Manson was the first to suggest that malaria might be spread by mosquitos. Finley embarked on a study of yellow fever, and after years of observations and experimentation he presented his findings to a conference in 1894 in which he advocated the eradication of the mosquito vectors.

Dr. Finley's recommendation was ignored. But the idea that mosquitos might be the culprit attracted the attention of Captain **Walter Reed** (1891-

1902), a U.S. Army surgeon. Reed had obtained a medical degree at the University of Virginia in 1869, and a second degree from Bellevue Medical School in New York. He joined the Army Medical Corp in 1874. He had made a specialty of bacteriology and was appointed professor of bacteriology at the Army Medical School. During the Spanish-American War he was appointed to head a commission to study the cause and spread of typhoid fever, one of the diseases that caused many of the American fatalities during this war. But it was apparent that yellow fever was the most dreaded disease that affected American troops. In 1897 Reed had been able to prove that the cause of yellow fever was not a bacterium as widely thought.

In 1899, after the war, Reed was made head of a commission to travel to Cuba to further investigate the disease. He concluded that the disease was not transmitted by bedding, clothing, or body contact. He turned to the idea already advanced by Finley that mosquitos are the culprits. Because there was no way of testing the idea on animals, there followed experiments in which some of the doctors of the commission allowed themselves to be bitten by mosquitos that had fed on yellow fever patients. One of the doctors of Reed's commission, **James Carroll** (1854-1907), who doubted that mosquitos were involved, allowed himself to be bitten by a mosquito that had bitten yellow fever patients. Within a few days he came down with a severe case of yellow fever, but survived. Another of the commission doctors, **Jesse William Lazear** (1866-1900), had not intended to join the experiment but while taking a blood sample from a patient he noticed that a mosquito had landed on his arm. Instead of slapping it, he allowed it to feed. Six days later he died of yellow fever.

In 1901 Reed determined that the causative agent of yellow fever was a virus. A Dutch botanist, **Martinus Beijerinck**, had discovered in 1898 that tobacco mosaic is caused by what he called a filterable virus; *virus* is Latin for *poison*. Reed's finding was the first time a human disease was attributed to a virus. The last of yellow fever in the United States was the flare-up in New Orleans in 1905. Reed did not live to see it; he died of appendicitis in 1901. The Army's Walter Reed General Hospital in Washington was named in his honor, and in 1945 he was elected to the Hall of Fame for Great Americans.

Another player in the hunt for the cause of yellow fever was **William Crawford Gorgas** (1854-1920), an American army surgeon who was assigned to the yellow fever problem in Havana from 1898 to 1902. In a career that closely paralleled that of Reed, Gorgas obtained his medical degree from Bellevue in 1879 and entered the army in 1880. In collaboration with Finley, he also came to believe in the theory of mosquito transmission. Gorgas was a man of action. Reducing the mosquito population by cleaning up mosquito breeding places, he was able to greatly reduce the occurrence of yellow fever in Havana. He went on to achieve distinction in Panama during building of the canal.

Constructing the Panama Canal was a monumental accomplishment, now designated an International Historic Civil Engineering Landmark. Equally spectacular was the control of malaria, and especially yellow fever, diseases that were largely responsible for the failure of an earlier attempt by a French company to build the canal. After the California gold rush of 1849, a way to transport voyagers and freight across the narrow Panama Isthmus, about 28 miles across at its narrowest point, was seen as an urgent need, thereby eliminating the long, expensive, and perilous sail around the horn from the Atlantic to the Pacific coast. The idea had been thought of centuries earlier when **Vasco Nuñez de Balboa**, who was the first European to reach the Pacific Coast, dreamed of building a canal across the isthmus.

In the 1840s the United States and Great Britain quarreled over who would control a canal through Nicaragua. In 1846, Columbia, of which Panama was a province, signed a treaty with the United States, which agreed to guard all trade routes across Panama. In 1850, a business group from New York made an agreement with Columbia to build a railroad across the isthmus, and that was finished in 1855, linking Colón on the Atlantic side with Panama City on the Pacific side. It helped, but there was still need for a canal for the passage of ships especially to haul freight. In 1878 Columbia made a deal with a French entrepreneur to build a canal across Panama. He sold the franchise to a French company headed by **Ferdinand Marie de Lesseps** who had built the Suez Canal. Although well planned by de Lesseps, the French attempt was a disaster, beset with theft of funds by French financial interests, inadequate equipment, and failure to protect workers against malaria and yellow fever. After digging up 76,000,000 cubic yards of earth for the canal, the company went bankrupt. Meanwhile, in 1889 a group of United States businessmen began a canal across Nicaragua, but they soon ran out of money. The way was clear for the United States government to become engaged in canal building.

In 1903 the United States signed a new treaty with Columbia in which the United States would pay Columbia $10,000,000 plus $250,000 annual rent for use of the canal zone. But the Columbia legislature thought it was not enough money so refused to ratify the treaty. Then things happened quickly. On November 3, 1903, with encouragement from both the French and the United States, the Panamanians revolted and declared Panama independent of Columbia. The United States sent ships to Panama ostensibly to protect the railroad. U.S. marines landed and prevented Columbian troops from marching on the city of Panama, the center of the revolt. On November 6, 1903, the United States recognized the Republic of Panama and two weeks later signed a treaty with the Republic of Panama giving the United States permanent, exclusive use of a 10-mile-wide canal zone. A year later the United States bought the French property.

It was seen that the greatest obstacle to building the canal would be the diseases that gave the French so much grief. In 1904, Lt. Colonel **William C. Gorgas**, who had cleaned up the mosquito-borne diseases of Havana, was given the responsibility of doing the same, but much more difficult task, in Panama. At first, Gorgas' efforts were devoted mainly to draining swamps, clearing brush and cutting areas of grass that harbored mosquitos. By 1906, he had stopped yellow fever and wiped out the rats that, with their fleas, were a threat of bubonic plague, and by 1913 he had made progress in greatly reducing the malaria rate. Gorgas was made Surgeon General of the U.S. Army, and later became engaged in the fight against yellow fever in other parts of the world. In 1950 he was elected to membership in the Hall of Fame for Great Americans.

The main work on the canal was completed by 1914 when a ship owned by the Panama Railroad Company made the first complete trip through the canal. President Woodrow Wilson proclaimed the official opening on July 12, 1920.

CHAPTER 15

A LOUSY WAR

This is the true story of how lowly blood-sucking lice helped defeat the French army and dethrone Emperor **Napoleon Bonaparte** (1769-1821). Nearly a century later scientists discovered the link between lice and the microorganism that causes *typhus*, the devastating disease that disrupted Napoleon's army.

Not many people, today, ever heard of epidemic typhus, a louse-borne disease that was a scourge in most parts of the world as recently as the early 1900s and is still a threat. It ravaged populations of people during war, famine, and where people were grouped together in congested conditions, such as crowded living quarters or institutions. One description of the disease was "jail fever."

Typhus was most apt to flare up in epidemic proportions during wars, especially among troops who are often required by circumstances to be in close contact and with few if any chances to bathe or change clothing. The misery of civilian disruptions associated with crowding, lack of cleanliness, food shortages, and disease often led to more loss of life than combat. Observers estimated that 3,000,000 died from the disease during the Russian Revolution. During and following World War II, epidemics of typhus occurred in North Africa, Yugoslavia, Japan, and Korea. Typhus was common in Nazi concentration camps.

Typhus is caused by pathogens belonging to a group called *rickettsia*[1, 2] which are microscopic organisms that share some of the characteristics of both bacteria and viruses. (Named in honor of an American pathologist, **Howard Taylor Ricketts** (1871-1910) who died while working on typhus in Mexico). Ricketts graduated from the University of Nebraska in 1894. His family fortune had been wiped out in the panic of 1893 so he had to work his way through medical school, finally getting his medical degree in 1897 at Northwestern University. After getting further training in Europe he joined the faculty of the University of Chicago in 1902.

Smaller than bacteria, they resemble them in having cell walls, enzymes, use oxygen, and are susceptible to antibiotics. Like viruses, they can live and multiply only inside cells. *Rickettsia prowaziki*, the epidemic typhus pathogen, damages the walls and linings of the blood vessels, causing bleeding and skin rashes. The disease strikes with a sudden onset of fever, headache, and extreme fatigue. Rash appears on the 4th to 6th day. If untreated the disease is apt to be fatal, especially in those over 50 years of age.

The first to discover that typhus was transmitted from person to person by the body louse, *Pediculus humanus corporus*, was **Charles Jules Henri Nicolle** (1866-1936), a French physician. Nicolle obtained his medical degree in 1893 after which he joined the faculty of the medical school in Rouen where his father was a professor. In 1902 he was appointed director of the Pasteur Institute in the colonial area of Tunis where he had an opportunity to study typhus. He had acquired an early interest in microbiology from a course that he had taken during his education.[3]

Nicolle noticed a strange thing about the typhus. It was very contagious among people generally, as well as among doctors who visited patients and also hospital employees who admitted patients. But after the patients were cleaned up, bathed, and their clothing washed, their ailment was no longer contagious. Since most of the patients were lousy when they arrived, Nicolle suspected that the body louse was the carrier, and in 1909 proved his conjecture by conducting experiments on animals, first chimpanzees, then guinea pigs. It was already known that mosquitoes transmit the pathogens of malaria and other diseases, so it was not surprising that the body louse was a transmitter. Nicolle never found the disease to be transferred from person to person directly in the absence of the insect carrier but it is now believed to be possible by contact with feces of infected lice.

Different species of rickettsia live in lice, fleas, mites, and ticks—all blood suckers. The one that lives in the body louse, *Pediculus humanus corporis*, is passed from person to person mostly by louse feces gaining entry through bites or other wounds.[4]

Nicolle observed that if animals succumbed to the disease and recovered, they might continue to carry the disease in mild form, or even without symptoms, but they could remain infective. It is possibly one explanation of how pathogens can persist without detection between epidemics and flare up again at a later time.

Typhus struck in midwinter of Napoleon's attempt to conquer Russia in 1812. During the retreat from Moscow, the combination of disease, bitterly cold weather, and harassment of the retreating troops caused terrible loss of life. Napoleon, known early in his career as *le petite Caporal* (the little corporal), demonstrated remarkable skill in handling and maneuvering troops. Soldiers under his command idolized him. His planning and management skills led to his rapid advancement to the rank of general. After defeating and controlling most of western and central Europe, he and his supporters seized power of the government of France in what was called the *Coup d' État* on November 9, 1799. The former little corporal then became dictator of France. In May in 1804 the French Senate voted him the title of Emperor.[5]

In 1807 Napoleon extracted an agreement with Czar **Alexander of Russia** to quit doing business with England, his enemy. Unhappy with the Czar's failure to close his ports to British trade, Napoleon decided to teach him a lesson. He conscripted an army of 600,000 men, many of them from countries under his control, and in the spring of 1812 marched them eastward across the steppes toward Moscow. The Russians resisted valiantly and retreated slowly, destroying everything of value and laid waste the countryside as they withdrew. Deprived of the usual war booty, the French troops' rations were limited, and when typhus struck they had to build makeshift hospitals from available debris. Napoleon pushed on to Moscow where to his surprise and deep disappointment, most of the people had left. The few remaining set fire to the city and left it in ruins.

After unsuccessfully trying to make a truce with the Czar, Napoleon had no choice but to turn back in retreat into the snow storms of a bitterly cold Russian winter. Troops were attacked by Cossacks especially at river crossings. The men were tired and weak from lack of food. Many were disabled from disease and extreme cold. Typhus took its toll. Accounts differ on how many lives were lost. A credible report said that 90,000 (15 per cent) made it back. If so, 510,000 did not survive (some were killed in battle or captured and a small few may have managed to escape into the wilderness).

It was the beginning of the end of Napoleon's empire. He turned command over to a general and hurried to Paris hoping to recruit a new army before word got out about his debacle. But it was too late. The news had spread, giving hope to conquered countries who made powerful alliances. He made several attempts to reassert his power but lost control in the gathering storm of his enemies. The French recalled Louis XVIII and crowned him king. Napoleon fought on, and when finally defeated by the British in the Battle of Waterloo, he tried to escape to America but was captured by the British and exiled to the small barren island of Saint Helena off the west coast of Africa where he died after a troubled illness on May 25, 1821, at the age of 52.

DEFEAT OF THE LICE

American soldiers in France during the World War (WWI) called body lice "cooties." Letters from the front often mentioned cooties because being bitten by them is not a pleasant experience. It causes a very annoying itch called pediculosis, and may result in systemic disturbances such as general feeling of tiredness, an irritable state of mind, loss of sleep, and a rash especially over the shoulders and abdomen. Continuous infestation causes a person's skin to harden and to become deeply pigmented, a condition referred to as "vagabond disease." Body lice prefer to hide out in clothing, especially where they are apt to be in close contact with the skin such as the crotch, armpits, waistline, neck, and shoulders. If present, they are always in underclothing but the eggs, called nits, were usually in the seams of the breeches.

Army medical authorities were well aware of the work of Nicolle and Ricketts on the relationship between body lice and typhus. They dealt with the threat by establishing delousing units that used sealed chambers, preferably with vacuum, to decontaminate clothing, and bedding if any, by fumigation with cyanide gas. While that was going on the soldiers would bathe and clean up. The most effective method was to use steam sterilization where steam was available. Steam is both "disinfecting and disinfecting." **William B. Herms**, an entomologist serving in the Medical Service Corp said that where fixed delousing stations were not available he organized a number of temporary stations using portable sterilizers. He "….arranged them in pairs side by side, each pair adjacent to a latrine with bath, one being used for blankets and underwear and the other for uniforms. About 35 men were handled per load every 30 to 35 minutes. Each station was in charge of a commissioned officer and five or six enlisted men as assistants."6

Delousing offered a quick means of lice destruction but its effectiveness had limitations. Fumigation kills the lice but not the nits (eggs), so the procedure had to be repeated frequently, and steam sterilizations usually required fixed equipment not readily transportable. Even portable sterilizers were not practical at the front.

It was not until the early stages of WWII that the body louse and its rickettsia surrendered—to a Swiss chemist, **Paul Hermann Müller** (1899-1965). Müller became a practicing chemist before returning to school at The University of Basel for his degree. He obtained his doctorate in 1925 after which he worked for a Swiss Dye company where in 1935 he began a research project to find a material that would kill insects quickly and safely. The insecticides then on the market either evaporated or disintegrated quickly or had to be eaten by the insects to kill them. Worse yet, the most commonly used insecticides on fruits and vegetables contained arsenic or lead, or both, or a fluoride. They often left poisonous residues on fruits and vegetables that were hard to wash off and it was not always done properly. The orchardist's dilemma was that without the protection of an insecticide the crop could be ruined by the feeding of insects or their larvae. "Wormy" apples and pears had little chance of bringing repeat customers.

Müller screened a large number of chemicals, looking for any that would be cheap, stable, without disagreeable odor, and of low toxicity to mammals, especially humans. The most promising ones that he screened contained chlorine, an ingredient of common salt (sodium chloride). In September of 1939 he synthesized and tried a compound described in chemical terms dichlorodiphenyltrichloroethane (DDT). It had been synthesized in 1873 by an earlier chemist who saved the sample as a curiosity. Müller tested it and found it to be remarkably effective and lacking the dangerous properties of lead, arsenic and others in common use.

The Swiss company put DDT on the market at once to control the Colorado potato beetle, a pest that by then had invaded Europe. United States manufacturers began producing the product in 1942. Although the initial use of DDT was against agricultural pests, it turned out that the effectiveness of DDT in preventing human diseases that are transmitted by insects was the greater discovery. In contrast to the commonly used inorganic poisons that were lethal to mammals, including humans, DDT was not only more effective against insects, it was less dangerous to use.

The value of a substance that is cheap, stable and low in toxicity to humans, and could be used to protect people from disease, was first demonstrated in Italy during WWII. When the American forces arrived in Sicily, dictator **Benito Mussolini** (1883-1945) who liked to be called *Il Duce* (the leader) was forced to resign and was imprisoned by the Italians for his disastrous effort to support Hitler's war of conquest. Mussolini's army had been defeated in North Africa, Ethiopia, and Eritrea. When German paratroopers arrived, they helped Mussolini escape from jail. He tried to flee to Switzerland with his mistress but they were captured by Italian pursuers and shot. Their bodies were brought to Milan and hung by their heels in front of a garage.

On the day the Allied forces landed on the Italian peninsula, October 13, 1943, Italy declared war on Germany. The American troops were confronted with an incipient epidemic of typhus in Naples. The army doctors asked for a supply of the new insecticide, DDT, which was rushed to Naples where DDT powder was blown onto the skin of millions of people including children. The epidemic was prevented and there were no reports of adverse effects.

Paul Müller was awarded the Nobel Prize in medicine and physiology in 1948 for his contribution to public health and nutrition. After the typhus episode in Italy, DDT was used to control malaria in Africa where it was so effective that it had the prospect of obliterating a disease that was killing, and still kills, nearly a million people each year. Why control of the disease did not actually happen is told in chapter 13.

CHAPTER 16

PLAGUES AND *THE PLAGUE*

Plagues, epidemics, and pandemics provide a window into the state of healing when outbreaks of the diseases afflicted humanity in earlier times. The term "plague" was used loosely to mean a disastrous epidemic. In that sense plagues ravaged people repeatedly for thousands of years.

The Book of Exodus describes ten plagues of Egypt. Among them: lice infested man and beast…all the cattle of the Egyptians died…an epidemic of boils afflicted men and animals…all the firstborn children and all the firstborn cattle of the Egyptians died (Israelite children were spared). The plagues were invoked on the Egyptians by **Moses** with the help of his brother **Aaron** who had supernatural powers. Moses and Aaron had previously tried to impress Pharaoh by turning a rod into a serpent, but Pharaoh scornfully turned it away as a parlor trick and asked his magicians to duplicate it, which they did.

Although the ten plagues of Egypt are depicted in the Book of Exodus as major catastrophes, there is no mention of them anywhere except in the Bible. But documented plagues were common in ancient times throughout the civilized world. **Homer** wrote in the *Iliad* of the gods inflicting people with plagues. The poem opens with a plague brought down on the people by **Apollo**. **Thucydides** wrote of a devastating epidemic, possibly smallpox, called the "Great Plague of Athens," that struck the city in 430-427 BC. It may have been the one that **Hippocrates** was credited with controlling and, if so, it was a major accomplishment because the most popular remedy in those days was to appeal to the gods for relief.

A plague, which also may have been smallpox, struck the Roman Empire in AD 165. The weary Romans were further weakened in 167 by a full scale military attack by the barbarians from the north. Still another epidemic hit enfeebled Rome in 262 killing, it is said, 5,000 people a day.

The Roman Empire had reached its peak of glory in the time of **Trajan** (98-117). The Empire then extended from the shores of the Caspian Sea in the east to the Atlantic coast of Spain in the west, and from Britain in the north to Egypt in the south. The vast expanse included hundreds of miles of roads and fortifications. Rome had become the largest city in the world, estimated to have at least a million, possibly a million and a half people. After the death of **Marcus Aurelius** in 180 the story of Rome is one of a long decline and fall, culminating in a split of the Empire. By the end of the fourth century during the reign of **Honorarius** (395-423) the Empire had become permanently split between east and west, with **Justinian** (527-565), the last of the great Emperors, holding forth in Constantinople where the disease, now simply called "Plague", hit the Mediterranean area.[1]

Plague is a medical term referring specifically to bubonic plague and related forms, a disease of such enormous devastation and suffering during the Middle Ages that it came closer than any other known natural event to wiping out civilization or even the possibility of the extinction of the human species. Plague, which still exists as an endemic disease of both people and rodents, can be transmitted to humans from the wild and for that reason health authorities keep a close watch over the possibility of outbreaks of the disease.[2]

Plague is caused by the bacterium *Yersinia pestis* (formerly known as *Pasterurella pestis*) which generally is acquired by being bitten by Oriental rat fleas *Xenopsylla Cheopis* which carry the bacterium from diseased, dying, or dead rats, mainly the so-called black rat, *Rattus rattus*, probably originally a native of Asia that infests houses, warehouses, and dwellings of all kinds throughout the world. It is also called the "ship rat" because it commonly hitches a ride as a stowaway aboard freighters. When a rat dies from the disease and turns cold, the fleas take off in search of a new source of warm blood, preferably a rat, but a sweaty sailor, stevedore, or passerby, will do. Upon the arrival of a ship in port, the rats with their flea population tend to get ashore as soon as the ship's hawsers are secured. Such immigrant pests and their germs typically thrive in coastal cities. The rats are called *reservoirs* of the disease, and fleas the *vectors*.

When an infected flea bites a person, some of the flea's saliva, along with its cargo of germs, gets into the wound, typically goes into the lymphatic system where the bacillus ends up in a lymph node. A large swelling or "bubo" develops at the site, hence the name bubonic plague. Buboes, typically in the lymph glands of the groin, armpits, or neck, range in size from 2 cm to 10 cm in diameter. This form of the disease resulted in about a 60 percent death rate. Another form of the disease, called the septicaemic form, is a result of the bacillus being injected by the flea directly into the blood stream. It is said to have been almost always fatal. Still another form of the disease, called pneumonic plague, could be transmitted from person to person directly without the insect vector. It, also, was almost always fatal.

It was not until the Plague epidemic had nearly played out after 12 centuries of disrupting civilized life that scientists made breakthrough discoveries of the cause of the disease. In 1897, **M. Ogata** infected mice with the plague bacterium by injecting them with an emulsion of crushed fleas that he took from plague infected rats. He reasoned that fleas must be the agents for natural transmission of the disease. He pointed out that fleas leave the dead rats as soon as they get cold and will seek another victim. They would no doubt prefer another rat but will settle for warm human blood. Then in 1898 a French scientist, **P. L. Simond**, succeeded in transmitting plague from a sick rat to a healthy rat by fleas.[3] Simond's results were not believed, but his finding was verified by **D. T. Verjbitski** who published his work in 1908.[4]

The original home of plague is believed to be the mountainous region of Central Asia, consisting of portions of Siberia, Mongolia, Tibet, and Manchuria. During an epidemic of the plague in Manchuria in 1910-1911 there were 60 thousand deaths from pneumonic plague. It is believed originally to have been spread to the human population by the tarbagan, *Arctomys bobac*, also known as the Siberian marmot, a large rodent about a half meter in length with a bushy tail about 15 cm long. It is a game animal sought by local hunters. The low body temperature during hibernation in the cold climate enables a diseased animal to survive, along with its fleas, and carry the infection over from one season to the next. Thus, the wild tarbagan, and its flea parasites are believed to serve as a reservoir of the disease, which could account for the persistently endemic nature of the plague in that part of the world.[5]

Germs were a lurking danger to our remote ancestors who lived in roving bands on the verge of becoming human. But it was not until people discovered the benefits of agriculture and industry, offering advantages of congregating in settlements, ultimately cities, that they became highly vulnerable to the calamity of epidemic diseases. The crowding of people increased transmission of germs and parasites. Congestion created hazardous sanitation conditions, accumulation of human waste, flies, vermin, and filth, contaminating water, food, and living quarters. In short, plagues were diseases of civilization (from the Latin word for "city dweller").

At the time of the great epidemics of plague, the size and congestion of the big cities had created conditions inimical to health. Garbage was dumped in backyards or ditches if they were handy. Human waste was thrown into the gutter to be washed away in rain water if it came. Sewer systems, if any, consisted of ditches alongside the roads, trash was sometimes deposited in a central pile in the middle of the city, and drinking water was from random sources sometimes from wells alongside outhouses. Conditions were made to order for flies and myriad other insects and vermin. Bathing was infrequent if it happened at all, and clothing was seldom washed, leaving a situation inviting the buildup and transmission of germs, parasitic worms, and insects. The man-made environment was one in which rats, flies, fleas, and lice could thrive. Epidemics of various kinds were inevitable. Forgotten were the sanitation practices of the Romans who constructed hundreds of miles of aqueducts to bring fresh water to the cities, luxuriated in heated baths, and built both private and public latrines with a system to flush away the waste.

A disastrous condition tied to the Plague that people could do nothing about, was a change in climate. The so-called Little Ice Age lasted from 1350 to 1870 in a sudden cold period following what is called the Little Climatic Optimum. During the 500-year period of the Little Ice Age when glaciers and ice caps expanded, the range of trees and other plants changed from where they could no longer exist to where they could survive. The ranges of animals that depended on certain plants, or on a milder climate, changed. Winters were colder and longer, summers were cooler and shorter, and precipitation was greater. The effect on agriculture was devastating. For example, crops such as the grains that once thrived in England could no longer mature during the short growing season. Shortages of food caused starvation, illness, and weakened conditions of people who would more easily succumb to diseases.[6]

The first recorded appearance of bubonic plague was in Egypt in AD 540. By AD 542 it had reached Constantinople where it is referred to as the Justinian Plague, so-called because it occurred during the reign of Emperor **Justinian** (527-565). It was said to have killed 10,000 people each day. By the time it subsided over 40 percent of the people had died. Plague spread throughout the eastern Mediterranean and was reported to have killed a fourth of the population. It spread further into Western Europe where episodes of the disease continued for two centuries before this wave of the disease faded. During the Great Plague of London in 1665 nothing was known about the cause of Plague although there was much speculation about humors, sick blood, and the wrath of gods. It would be another 1,200 years after the calamity of the Black Death in Europe, before studies by investigators during the Scientific Revolution would unravel the puzzle and reveal the triple threat of rats, fleas and bacteria.[7]

The time between the great "plague" of Athens in 430 BC during the Golden Age of Greece and the Justinian Plague (bubonic plague) in AD 542, the decline of the Roman Empire was a long period of sustained political upheaval in the Mediterranean world. When the Peloponnesian War weakened Athens and the other cities it quarreled with, leading to the takeover of Greece by the Macedonian king, **Philip**, and his son, **Alexander**, Rome was a small city of little importance still engaged in repulsing sporadic attacks from barbarian tribes in the north. But along with the slow decline of Greek influence, the power of Rome spread throughout the Mediterranean area and beyond.

A virulent form of the Plague, and the most devastating episode of the disease, referred to as the Black Death—the Germans called it the Great Dying—originated in Asia where it apparently had been endemic. The disease moved in a westward path into the Crimea in 1343 where Genoese traders were infected. They managed to sail their ship back to Italy with everyone on board dead or dying. The disease, having engulfed Constantinople by 1347, surged westward blanketing the Mediterranean area and overwhelming western Europe in an epidemic of sudden death, leaving people in a chaotic state of fear, panic, and despair. It killed off at least a fourth of the population of western Europe during the three years of its lethal attack. Between 1334 and 1351, the plague spread through Italy, France, England, Germany, Norway, Russia, India, Persia, and China. The Roman Empire had reportedly already lost a fourth of its population to the disease during the so-called Justinian Plague. By December 1348 the Black Death had reached the northern part of the British Isles. It is estimated that the first wave of Black Death between 1347 and 1350 had killed 20 million people in Europe alone. Following the original devastation, the disease struck in sporadic attacks for the next two centuries, then dwindled to what appeared to be occasional new introductions from Asia until 1800.

Black Death was a disease that killed quickly, often within a day of the first symptoms. The disaster was unprecedented and beyond imagination. It is believed that it killed one third of the human population worldwide. No one had any idea of the cause of the disease or how to treat it. Simple hygiene such as body cleanliness, bathing, clean clothing, and disposal of waste and trash that could provide cover for rats and insects were at best only for the affluent. The only defense was flight from the city by those who had country estates or otherwise could afford it. Florence was not only a major city, it suffered havoc as bad, perhaps worse, than any other European big city. A reasonably accurate estimate is that Florence lost three-quarters of its population between 1338 and 1447.[8] Death and desolation were so frightful that the citizens of Florence prohibited entry of sick people into the city. (See quarantine)

The *Decameron*, by **Geovanni Boccaccio** (1313-1375), is a collection of 100 short lively tales that were supposed to have been told to a group of revel-making cavaliers and maidens who had fled the plague in Florence to take refuge in a country house. Boccaccio gave an eyewitness account of the chaotic devastation in Florence in the preamble of the *Decameron*.[9]

The Great Plague of London in 1665 extending over a three year period (1664-1666) was immortalized by Daniel Defoe (c.1660-1731) in a fictionalized account, *A Journal of the Plague Year*, which might pass as a documentary by later journalistic standards.[10] It is reliably estimated that in London 70,000 people died out of a population of 450,000. In all of Great Britain from half to two-thirds of the people perished.

During the worst of the epidemics of Plague in such cities as Florence and London, taking care of the sick, dying, and dead was a chaotic nightmare beyond compare. People died in the streets and lay in the gutters to be picked up and carted away. Corpses were stacked onto wagons and hauled away to common graves. Worst of all, there were people who fled their houses, leaving the sick and dying, sometimes children, to care for themselves.

People who knew nothing about the cause of an epidemic had a sense that the disease could be caught by being with or by touching those who were sick with it. During the black plague in England, many of the dying were left at home alive, and often the dead were shoved into a roadside ditch or hauled away in wagons to be buried in common unmarked graves. In 1403, Venice prevented strangers from entering the city until they had waited outside for a specified time to see if they were free of the dreaded disease before being permitted to enter. It was decided that the waiting time should be set at forty days, possibly influenced by the forty day periods mentioned in the Bible. The waiting period for Venice was called *quarantine*, from the French word for "forty." It was the first known action in public hygiene taken by a government agency.[10]

The plague mysteriously disappeared from most parts of Europe, possibly in part due to the displacement of the black rat by the local brown rat, also known as the wharf or sewer rat, *Rattus norvegicus*. However, a third outbreak of plague broke out in China. As recently as 1894 it appeared in Hong Kong and spread to other parts of the world. During the next 20 years more than 10 million people died from the plague in India. It is speculated that the India pandemic also originated in tarbagan (*Arctomys bobac*), a wild rodent that thrives in the interior of China. The wave surged eastward, moving into Australia and the west coast of the United States where it struck San Francisco in an incipient epidemic in 1900. At that point, although the plague remained endemic in Asia, the feared pandemic in the New World fizzled out. Reasons are speculative. What we do know is that a timely breakthrough in medical science made it possible for a hygienic attack on the disease and to eradicate the cause.

When plague showed up in San Francisco in 1900, authorities had the advantage of being alerted to the role of rats and fleas in transmission of the disease. A vigorous campaign against the rats by poisoning, fumigation, and trapping was followed. The so-called ship rat, or black rat, *Rattus rattus*, knew its way around the world. Whenever a ship tied up at a wharf, some of the stowaway rats would come ashore by traveling down the hawser lines to the wharf. It was possible to thwart the rat in its attempt to board ship or debark by attaching metal cones on the hawsers. Rats trying to get up or down the line were apt to lose their footing and fall into the water.

Since plague is essentially a rodent disease, it was no surprise that it spread to ground squirrels. Several people acquired bubonic plague before experiments showed it to be the same disease in humans and squirrels and that it could be transmitted by fleas, of which several species infest squirrels. Plague remains endemic in squirrels today, so public health workers remain alert to reports of dead or sick squirrels because there is danger of transmission to residents and especially vacationers in parks and mountain areas wherever the ubiquitous squirrels thrive.

Ranchers hit on the idea of killing squirrels and other rodents by spreading the disease among them by tossing plague-killed squirrels along with their fleas into their nests. It was not very practical because other methods are more efficient. Anyway, biological warfare was not original with the ranchers. Warring factions in the Middle Ages tried various schemes. One was to pollute the enemy's water supply. Another was during the outbreak of the Black Death when war broke out between the Tartars and the Italian merchants in the Crimea, the Christians withdrew to the citadel at Kaffa where the Tartars put them under siege. Plague forced the Tartars to withdraw but before doing so, they catapulted the bodies of plague victims over the walls.[11] And during the war against the American Indians, United States troops gave them blankets taken from victims of smallpox, with disastrous results to the Indians who had no natural immunity to the disease.

Plague has flared up sporadically in various parts of the world in modern times but vigorous public health measures to control the rats and flea vectors have kept the bacterium within bounds in most places.

PART IV
DRUGS

17 WONDER DRUGS

18 MAD MICROBES

19 RIGHT AND LEFT OF MEDICINES

20 FDA: 300-YEAR WAR

21 CHINESE PUZZLE

22 A BLOODY SHAME

CHAPTER 17

WONDER DRUGS

A new era in medicines came with the discovery of the antibiotics. Important work by microbiologists beginning early in the twentieth century led to what we enjoy now as an arsenal of dozens of antibiotics with a variety of applications against infections. The discovery of antibiotics was the culmination of many preliminary developments by talented researchers. An important contributor was **Paul Ehrlich** (1854-1915), a German bacteriologist. The son of a prosperous Jewish businessman, Ehrlich did poorly in school but he developed an interest in both biology and chemistry which he made a point of combining in medical school, unusual for a budding scientist in those days. He took an interest in the new aniline dyes and their use in staining cells and microbes. He found that a dye stained some kinds of cells and not others. He reasoned that if a microbe took the color there was a reaction taking place and incidentally discovered that a dye called Tripan Red inhibited the growth and development of the trypanosome that causes sleeping sickness.

After obtaining his medical degree at Leipzig in 1878 he found a way to stain the tubercle bacillus which brought him to the attention of the German bacteriologist **Robert Koch** (1843-1910) who had made a specialty of tuberculosis. Ehrlich worked with Koch but after acquiring a mild case of tuberculosis he retired to Egypt where he hoped the mild climate would cure him, which it did. Upon his return he joined forces with two bacteriologists who had worked with Koch, **Emil Behring** (1854-1917) and **Baron Kitasato** (1856-1931) who were trying to find a cure for diphtheria by producing antibodies in animals inoculated with the diphtheria germ. In 1892 they produced an antitoxin that was wonderfully successful. The work earned Ehrlich a professorship at the University of

Berlin and for Behring the first Nobel Prize ever in medicine and physiology.

Ehrlich's major fame came from establishing a method for screening hundreds of chemicals in search of the "magic bullet" against microorganisms. He had noticed the similarity between the chemical reactions of hydrogen and those of arsenic, so most of the compounds in his trials were arsenicals.

He hit the jackpot with the 606th that an assistant found remarkably effective against the spirochete that causes syphilis, a dreaded, almost secret disease. By then Ehrlich was testing in the 900s. At first he called the medicine 606 then named it Salvarsan, the first effective and relatively safe medicine for the cure of syphilis. Salvarsan is now known by its short chemical name arsphenamine. In 1908 Ehrlich was awarded a share of the Nobel Prize in Medicine and Physiology, along with a Russian-French bacteriologist **Ilya Mechnikov** (1845-1916) for his work on white corpuscles at the Pasteur Institute.

Ehrlich's work from trypan red to salvarsan marked the beginning of an era in modern *chemotherapy*, a word coined by Ehrlich. Actually, chemicals had been used much earlier for the treatment of diseases, for example quinine for malaria, foxglove for heart disease, cantharides from the Spanish fly for "blistering," and several toxic minerals, but Erhlich's chemotherapy as envisioned by him had to wait for the systematic research of the pharmacology industry.

Meanwhile, a forerunner to the mainstream antibiotics was the work of **Gerhard Domagk** (1895-1964), a German biochemist. The son of a teacher, Domagk had barely started his education at the University of Kiel when World War I prompted him to volunteer. He was wounded in 1915 and was transferred to the Medical Corp. After the war, he returned to the university where he obtained a medical degree. Enticed by industry, he went to work for I. G. Farbenindustrie, a firm that pioneered making synthetic dyes. Domagk conducted a systematic survey of dyes for the purpose of finding biological activity that might have medical applications. One of the new products, an orange-red dye with the trade name Prontosil, when injected into mice greatly reduced the infection from the bacterium *Streptococcus*. It was an important discovery because none of the previously introduced medications had any effect on the most common forms of bacteria causing infection.

Domagk demonstrated the effectiveness of Protosil in a dramatic way. His daughter, **Hildegarde**, became infected with streptococci from the prick of a needle. Nothing did any good until Domagk in desperation injected a large amount of Prontosil. The story of her recovery helped spread the word around the world in 1935 of a new powerful drug. Its fame was further enhanced when it was used to save the life of **Franklin D. Roosevelt, Jr.**, son of the president of the United States. Domagk was awarded the Nobel Prize in medicine and physiology in 1939 for his discovery. Hitler was in a rage over the committee's award of the Nobel Prize for peace to **Karl von Ossietzky**, a German pacifist in a concentration camp. He refused to allow any German to accept a Nobel Prize. So Domagk had to wait until after the war and Hitler was dead to visit Stockholm to accept the Nobel Prize, although award of the money had expired.

Daniele Bovet (1907-1992), a Swiss-French-Italian pharmacologist, took an interest in a strange feature of Prontosil. Bovet, the son of a professor of pedagogy, received his doctorate from the University of Geneva in 1929 and engaged in work at the Pasteur Institute in Paris. He and his colleagues observed that Prontosil, though effective against *Streptococcus* in the body, had no effect on the bacteria in a test tube. They reasoned that Prontosil must be an innocuous chemical that has to be changed in the body to something else that will kill bacteria. The most obvious change would be for the chemical to break up into two or more of its parts. One of the parts, sulfanilamide, which they tested at the Pasteur Institute in 1936, proved to be effective in both the body and in a test tube. It led to the array of "sulfa" drugs that were important in treating wounds during the World War II years and for civilian use as well.

Later studies determined what made sulfanilamide and the other sulfa drugs such good bacteria killers. An enzyme that occurs naturally in the bacteria has the function of reacting with para-aminobenzoic acid (PABA) which it uses as a precursor of the needed vitamin folic acid. Unfortunately for the bacteria, the enzyme just as readily attacks sulfanilamide, which is similar in chemical structure to, and easily mistaken for, PABA. In the presence of sulfanilamide the enzyme supply is quickly used up, leaving no way for the PABA to be utilized in making folic acid. Species of bacteria that do not need folic acid or those that can obtain it from extraneous sources are not killed by sulfa drugs. Nor do the sulfa drugs adversely affect humans or other animals. We do not need to synthesize folic acid. We get it in our diet.

Bovet made several other discoveries that were therapeutically important, and was awarded the 1957 Nobel Prize for medicine and physiology.

Meanwhile others were engaged in studies that might lead to control of infections. **Selman Abraham Waksman** (1888-1973), a Russian microbiologist, took an interest in microorganisms found in the soil. Waksman arrived in the United States in 1910, attended Rutgers University, graduating in 1915 and became an American citizen a year later. After obtaining his doctorate at the University of California in 1918 he returned to Rutgers as a member of the faculty. In his search for substances in microorganisms that would kill bacteria, Waksman coined the name "antibiotic" for such chemicals. He had studied *Streptomyces* molds since starting his graduate work and finally in 1943 he isolated an antibiotic that he named Streptomycin, effective against gram-negative bacteria, named after **Hans Christian Joachim Gram** (1853-1938) who made discoveries of how bacteria take different stains. Gram-negative bacteria have a tough outer coat that makes them generally highly resistant to antibiotics. Streptomycin was first marketed in 1945. For his discovery, Waksman was awarded the 1952 Nobel Prize for medicine and physiology.

René Jules Dubos (1901- 1982), a graduate student of Waksman, had studied agricultural sciences in France and arrived in America in 1924. He obtained his doctorate at Rutgers where, under the influence of Waksman, he studied soil microorganisms and was interested in finding antibacterial chemicals in them. He joined the Rockefeller Institute for Medical Research (later Rockefeller University) where he isolated a mixture of substances that he called tyrothricin. It did not become a very successful pharmaceutical but Dubos and his work were influential in stimulating an interest in the search for and developing uses for antibiotics, including penicillin.

A key figure in the discovery of the remarkable effects of antibiotics was **Alexander Fleming** (1881-1955), a Scottish bacteriologist, who was the first to detect the spectacular antimicrobial effect of *penicillin*. He was the seventh of eight children in a farm family whose father died when Alexander was quite young. They had little money so Alexander went to London where he found work as a shipping clerk, then he joined the army during the Boer war but not soon enough to see service before the war ended in 1902. That year he received a scholarship which, with a legacy from an uncle, enabled him to begin medical studies at the University of London, where he received his medical degree in 1906. He served in the medical corps of the British army during World War I, and after the war he obtained an appointment as professor at the Royal College of Surgeons, where he developed an interest in bacteriology, especially in chemicals for control of diseases. In 1928, he returned to the University of London where he had been a medical student and was appointed professor of bacteriology.

Fleming's most important discovery came by accident in 1928, and as luck would have it, the result of what by today's laboratory standards would be called sloppy, even dangerous, technique. He had taken up work on *Staphylococcus aureus*, a notorious life-threatening cause of wound infections. After finishing with some cultures he tossed the plates into a tray, and after returning from a holiday while preparing to disinfect them, happened to pick up a plate that had an unusual growth in it. There was a large colony of mold around which there was a clear area with no *Staph* colonies. Fleming isolated the mold, cultured it and determined that it was *Penicillium notatum*, a mold similar to what you might find on stale bread. He surmised that the mold had released some chemical that inhibited bacterial growth, and whatever it was, called it penicillin. Fleming was not a chemist, so he did not further pursue its identity.

Fleming published his findings, but for reasons that are not clear, no one seemed to be excited about the most exciting discovery ever made in antimicrobials. But with the outbreak of World War II there was imminent need for remedies for infected wounds. Between 1939 and 1945 more than 9,000,000 allied service men died and about 6,000,000 from the axis countries were killed. At least three times that many were wounded. Domagk's Prontosil derivative sulfanilamide, introduced in 1935, was the mainstay for preventing infection of wounds, and Dubos' isolation of the first antibiotic, tyrothricin, in 1939 stimulated a search for more effective antibiotics.

Howard Walter Florey (1898-1968), an Australian-English pathologist, had been working on Fleming's antibacterial lysozyme. Florey had attended the University of Adelaide where he obtained his medical degree in 1921, then as a Rhodes Scholar, he studied at Oxford and Cambridge where he received a Ph.D. in 1927. He decided to work, in collaboration with **Ernst Boris Chain** (1906-1979), a German-English biochemist, on the active ingredient of Fleming's *Penicillium* mold. They soon obtained a yellow powder that contained a quantity of the antibiotic. Research on the product in both Great Britain and the United States succeeded in producing enough for trial use in 1943 (at last, 15 years after Fleming's discovery) to treat war casualties in Tunisia and Sicily. By 1945, a half ton a month was being made. The chemical structure was determined and methods for producing large quantities were devised. After the war penicillin's effectiveness combined with its low toxicity made it the most valuable of the antibiotics, its usefulness now lasting for decades.

Fleming was knighted in 1944, becoming Sir Alexander Fleming. Florey was knighted in 1944, elected president of the Royal Society, became provost of Queen's College, Oxford, and was given a life peerage, becoming Baron Florey of Adelaide. Fleming, Florey and Chain shared the 1945 Nobel Prize in medicine and physiology. (Florey's picture is on the Australian 50-pound note.)

CHAPTER 18

MAD MICROBES

It wasn't long after the introduction of the arsenal of miracle drugs—the antibiotics—that we became aware of impending trouble. Sometimes treatment failed to clear up the infection, making it necessary to switch to another antibiotic that might do the job. Microbes had responded with the perfect defense: resistance. In some cases bacteria became resistant to almost any antibiotic we could come up with. Resistant bacteria became almost epidemic in hospitals where, despite scrubbing and swabbing, microbes pass from person to person, often the result of poor hygiene. One of the worst is methicillin-resistant *Staphylococcus aureus* (MRSA) that kills thousands of patients annually, said to exceed the deaths from AIDS in the United States. MRSA is a major problem in hospitals requiring meticulous but often neglected, care and cleaning.[1]

An even more dangerous form of resistant bacteria is the air-borne *Mycobacterium tuberculosis* that causes one or more of the various forms of the debilitative disease tuberculosis (TB). Multi-drug resistance to tuberculosis (MDR-TB) has reached epidemic proportions in India, sometimes requiring repeated treatments with different drugs several times a year, often year after year for hopefully a cure. Tests show resistance to TB of seven drugs. The disease is not a trivial problem. India is believed to have nearly a fourth of the world's 8.7 million TB patients. An India government report stated that the resistance rate is probably much higher than the 2 to 3% reported to the World Health Organization (WHO). Their data from 18 sites showed 6.7% of TB patients were drug resistant. South Africa, another TB hot bed, reported that trials of a common form of resistance gave results in two hours instead of weeks or months.

Tuberculosis is an ancient affliction. During the Industrial Revolution when overcrowding was common, TB accounted for more than 30% of all deaths. With development of antibiotics in the 1940s and later, TB appeared to be under control. But it was never easy to cure. Diagnosis is difficult, often requiring repeated tests. When found to be present it must be treated. Otherwise about half of the infections will progress to full blown TB in the lung or another susceptible organ. Listed in the Merck Manual of Medical Information under the heading Tuberculosis, A Disease of Many Organs: Abdominal cavity, Bladder, Brain, Pericardium (the membranous sac around the heart), Joints, Kidney, Reproductive organs (men: lump in scrotum, women: Sterility), Spine.

Resistance in medicines used for treatment of tuberculosis (TB) has spread to several parts of the world. According to a study made by Geeta Anand, Shreya Shaw and Betsy McKay[2] India is home to a quarter of the world's TB patients totaling 8.8 million. The World Health Organization (WHO) gave the breakdown: India: 2.3 million, China: 1.0 million, Russia: 150.000, Brazil: 5.000, U.S.: 13.000.

Tuberculosis is caused by an infection with the bacterium, *Mycobacterium tuberculosis*, commonly acquired by inhaling air contaminated with the bacterium. In some countries children become infected with a related bacterium, *Mycobacterium bovis*, acquired by drinking unpasteurized milk.

The mycobacterium may linger for years in the lungs or other tissues of the body without the patient being aware of the infection. A common diagnostic procedure is the tuberculin skin test that can reveal a past infection. Often the first indication of active tuberculosis is an abnormal chest x-ray. The disease can usually be cured by the use of antibiotics. Because the tissues will contain thousands of bacteria, it is necessary to use at least two drugs having different methods of action and to continue treatment long after the patient feels completely well to avoid the chance that some of the slow-growing bacteria may cause a relapse.

It is not surprising that strains of *Mycobacterium* have developed multi-drug resistance. There are 17 drugs recommended by the World Health Organization (WHO) for TB treatment. They differ widely in effectiveness. Hopefully, some will remain useful against TB for years to come.

There was nothing new about biological resistance. All organisms in the world of nature are able to perpetuate their species despite the abundance of innumerable dangerous and toxic substances in the environment. During eons of survival, organisms acquired various physiological strategies to contend with toxins. In humans, and other higher animals, the liver is where the most active biochemical detoxification takes place—through enzymatic destruction of unwanted foreign substances.

Early in the last century we became aware of the ability of populations of organisms, that at first were highly susceptible, to develop resistance to chemicals intended to kill them. An early warning was when doctors found it more difficult to cure an infection of gonorrhea, caused by the bacterium *Neisseria gonorrhoeae* with the conventional treatment.

Insects resistant to poisons were among the first to be thoroughly studied. Apple farmers found that they had to increase the amount of chemical that was used at the time, lead arsenate, to suppress infestations of codling moth, the larvae of which caused "wormy" apples. Unfortunately neither wormy apples nor apples with a thick coat of poison were saleable. In 1916 the California red scale, *Aonidiella aurantii*, became resistant to fumigation with hydrogen cyanide. The red scale is a small insect that attaches itself in large numbers to leaves, stems, and fruits and subsists by sucking juice from tissues of the plant. The resistant scales slowly spread over a wide agricultural area and became so hard to kill that four to five times the original dose of the poison was required and the use of hydrogen cyanide had to be abandoned. Resistance of insects to poisons became common. A spectacular case was that of DDT-resistant houseflies, which evolved to produce greatly increased amounts of a detoxifying enzyme, dehydrochlorinase, that acts to convert the insecticide DDT to a nontoxic compound. Strains of laboratory flies became so resistant that they survived several hundred times the original lethal dose. In a study of another insecticide, dieldrin, resistance appeared to be due to a single gene.

Organisms have several biochemical and behavioral strategies to resist poisons. But the overriding force is Darwinian (natural) selection. All plants, animals, bacteria, or whatever organisms you might name, are subject to mutations, from large and lethal to almost insignificant, as a result of which members of the given population differ in characteristics. To name a few: size, weight, height, color, strength, health, smoothness, stamina, longevity. If, for example, you were to pick ten thousand men at random and measure their heights, some would be extremely tall and some extremely short but most would be lumped in between. Plotting the numbers against height gives the so-called bell curve, high in the middle and tailing off at the extreme ends. Many physiological conditions in a given population of organisms can be expected to follow a bell curve. Thousands of experimental tests with toxins show that a dose not quite high enough to kill all the organisms will leave naturally resistant mutants to reproduce the resistance characteristic.

In bacteria, a dose of super drug like an antibiotic will kill all of the susceptible bacteria but may leave a few that are resistant. The survivors will give rise to a new population of resistant bacteria.

So the mad microbes play the Darwin gig—*survival of the fittest*—despite enormous casualties. However, it is only a partial explanation of their antibacterial success. The have sex—the way they do it—as a weapon.

Single cell sex was no doubt an early innovation. The first living things to emerge from the tortured planet during the creation of life may have been sexless. But sex, that is, the transfer of genetic material from one organism to another, must have appeared soon because it exists in one form or another in the simplest of organisms. Even viruses, those tiny bundles of molecules in the twilight zone between the living and nonliving, have their special brand of sex.

Sex in the small world of microbes is a big cause of human misery. Sexually active bacteria are by nature promiscuous. They have several ways of passing their genes from one to another, although microbiologists do not consider all of such activity as actually sexual because transfer of cytoplasm may be involved instead. But microbes are adept at indiscriminately passing their genetic material on to others of their kind, or to others not exactly their kind.

The role of single cell sex in disease organisms was discovered in 1928 by **Frederick Griffith**, a British scientist working in the Pathological Laboratory of the Ministry of Health. He was working on *Streptococcus pneumoniae* (pneumococcus) bacterium that causes pneumonia. There are two different strains of the bacterium, one with a smooth carbohydrate coat (S), and the other lacking a coat and therefore having a rough appearance (R). When injected into mice, the S-type is highly infective whereas the R-type is harmless to humans, apparently because it has no carbohydrate coat to protect itself from counterattack by the human body's defenses.

The S-type bacteria have three variants depending on the kind of carbohydrate coat, designated I, II, and III. Griffith killed some S-type III bacteria with heat and injected some of the dead bacteria into mice, and at the same time, injected them with some living, harmless R-type bacteria. Surprisingly, all the mice died. Griffith determined that they contained living S-type III bacteria. The harmless R-type bacteria had become infective S-type bacteria! Can there be sex after death in the microbe world? Griffith went on to show that the transformation could be inherited. Although he was too shy to publicize his discovery, it was promptly confirmed by German scientists.

Two years later, a Canadian-American physician, **Oswald Avery** (1877-1955), at the Rockefeller Institute, now Rockefeller University, started work on pneumococci. He and his co-workers were able to transform living R-Type into S-type in a glass dish. They did it by culturing R-type bacteria in a filtered extract of killed S-type bacteria. The extract was effective at a concentration of one part in 600 million. Everyone thought that the mysterious extract must be an enzyme (a protein), but Avery and his associates found that the active substance was pure DNA. They reported the results in 1944.

Griffith and Avery had shown that genetic material of bacteria can be transferred to other organisms even after the death of the donor. Japanese scientists made a related discovery in 1959. They found that dysentery-causing bacteria could pass their genes for resistance to *E. Coli*, the common intestinal bacterium, and that *E. Coli* in turn can pass it to *Salmonella*, another troublesome intestinal pathogen. And in 1970, **Robert Ferone** and his co-workers were able to show that the malaria protozoan parasite, *Plasmodium,* can transfer resistance to the drug pyramethamine from one species of protozoan to another.

Headline scenario: *Man bites dog*. Not true. *Bacterium chows down on antibiotic.* True. **George Church**, a geneticist at Harvard Medical School and associates were looking for microbes that could make biofuels out of agricultural waste. They used antibiotics to make sure they had active organisms. But some of the bacteria they collected from soil made a meal of the antibiotics. Every sample that they collected from 11 different sites, from a cornfield to virgin forest, had bacteria that thrived on nothing but antibiotics. Every one of the medicines tested, including such commonly used antibiotics as penicillin and ciprofloxacin was chomped on by at least one type of bacteria. Said Church, "Almost all the drugs that we consider as our mainline defense against bacterial infections are at risk from bacteria that not only resist the drugs but eat them for breakfast."[3]

CHAPTER 19

RIGHT AND LEFT HAND OF MEDICINE

A characteristic of many animals, including us, is bilateral symmetry, that is, the same on both sides—two arms and hands, two legs and feet, two eyes, two ears, two nostrils, two lungs, two kidneys, two ovaries, two testicles, two of some other glands, and even right and left halves of the cerebral cortex. The redundancy of double endowment can be live saving. If one of the pair is injured, often the other can take over.

Some of the paired parts are mirror images of each other. The two hands look almost alike superficially, but they are opposites, and don't perform exactly alike. Even at the molecular level, many organic chemicals are formed as mirror images. But living systems are untrained in equal opportunity. They are almost always strongly biased toward one or the other mirror-image twin. One of the great mysteries of nature is why living systems consistently opt for one or the other of a pair of look-a-likes, or pick a particular one of two ways of doing things. Most people are right-handed (controlled by the left side of the brain); honeysuckle stems corkscrew around each other always in the same direction; snails and seashells always spiral one way or the other in the same species. At the submicroscopic level, even electrons spin one way or the other depending on their status in the atom.

Chemicals that exist in the two forms, called *isomers*, from the Greek *isomeres*, meaning "equally divided," can be compared to baseball players, some of whom are right-handed and some left-handed. There are no right-hand or left-hand baseballs and no right-hand or left-hand bats. But a right-hand glove will fit only a right-handed catcher and a left-hand glove will fit only a left-handed catcher. Molecules existing as mirror images relate to players in living systems in much the same way.

The property of handedness goes by the technical term "chirality", from the Greek *cheir*, meaning "hand." Thus, a substance that has handedness such as an amino acid, is said to be "chiral." Another way of saying it is that two mirror image chemicals are referred to as "enantiomers" from the Greek *enantios*, meaning opposite. A 50-50 mixture of enantiomers is said to be "racemic" from the Latin *racemus*, "a cluster of grapes." The most convenient way to describe comparative handedness is to refer to the way it twists light, for example, a left twisting molecule is a levo-molecule whereas a right twisting molecule would be a dextro-molecule.

Chirality is important in medicine. All natural amino acids, the building blocks of proteins, have the levo-configuration. Thus natural proteins are all L-proteins. It is important when the effect of a medicine is to react with another chemical.

Pasteur discovered that a mold used only one of two forms—left (*levo*) and right (*dextro*)—of molecules that he offered it.[1, 2, 3] The commercial importance of the biological selectivity of isomers became apparent early in the 20th century. It was long known that nicotine was a good insecticide. Tobacco "sweepings" from the manufacture of cigarettes were used either by grinding into a fine powder for dusting on plants, or by extracting the nicotine as a liquid for spraying in diluted form. Although small amounts of nicotine are highly poisonous to people as well as bugs, nicotine had the obvious virtue of disappearing from the plants quickly, usually within a few hours or at most a few days. Nicotine sulfate, sold under the trade name "Black Leaf 40", was available in seed and nursery stores and other commercial outlets (as recently as 1975, an estimated 500 tons of pure nicotine equivalent per year were produced in the United States).[4] Enterprising people of the chemical industry found that they could manufacture nicotine synthetically. With visions of capturing a large share of the profits in the nicotine market monopolized by the big tobacco companies, they proceeded to test the manufactured product on insects. To their surprise, they found that it was only half as effective as the natural product. The manufactured material was a 50-50 mixture of the left-handed and right-handed mirror images, so it contained only half as much of the toxic levo-nicotine as the natural nicotine, which is 100% left-handed (levo-) nicotine. The bugs could handle the right-handed dextro-nicotine with impunity, but were knocked out by the natural left-handed poison.

The handedness of many manufactured organic compounds that are used widely in modern life, has come to be of increasing interest in medicine. Pharmaceutical manufacturers are in search of ways to improve the potency or yield of chiral drugs by developing methods to produce a higher proportion of the active isomer. The United States Food and Drug Administration (FDA) is keeping a close look on these efforts to make sure that elimination of the presumably inactive form doesn't have some unrecognized effect. Many drugs are prescribed and administered at doses that are at or close to the borderline of serious side effects. Knowledge of the potency of individual doses is crucial. Manufacturers are also becoming keenly interested in chiral forms of flavors and fragrances.

You might think that the extensive use of left-handed molecules by living systems is proof that the Creator made a left turn when life began, and set that path as the way to go for the millions of generations that followed. But not so fast. Nature is full of twists and turns. A helix can be twisted to either the right or left, but in nature the double helix of DNA always twists to the right, comparable to the right-hand twist of a corkscrew, or a manmade screw which to be set has to be turned to the right, or the twist of threads on a bolt, the nut for which has to be turned to the right to tighten.

We already know that most of the sugars are right-handed, for example dextrose. But they play a role less extensive and probably far less ancient than the amino acids, powerful rulers behind the throne. The potentate of life, the right-twisted DNA, can't do much of anything by itself. Like the sound track on a film, it carries the code for the signal and like a conductor it waves the baton but doesn't play the music. To make the thousands of proteins used in a living system, DNA needs the help of its sidekick, RNA. To make a protein, a strand of RNA snuggles alongside one of the strands of DNA where it makes a complementary copy of a piece of the code, comparable to a negative image. Playing the role of so-called messenger RNA (mRNA), it carries the transcribed code to one of the structures in the cytoplasm of the cell called *ribosomes*. The ribosomes are microscopic, highly efficient, protein factories where appropriate three-letter pieces (codons) are translated back to their original genetic code by a form of RNA called transfer RNA (tRNA) which initiates assembly of the protein. The raw material used by the ribosomes consists of 20 kinds of amino acids, all chiral. There is tRNA for each of the amino acids; and they are all lefties.[5]

All proteins, including enzymes, in all living organisms that have been studied, have only left-handed amino acids. There are thousands of enzymes among the body's 60,000 or so proteins. But there is no known natural law that would prevent proteins from using right-handed amino acids. **Stephen Kent** and his associates at the Scripps Research Institute synthesized an opposite-handed enzyme—containing all right-handed amino acids.[6] Not long ago, the idea of life on other worlds was the domain of science fiction, but now extraterrestrial life is a serious scientific study. Beyond other worlds, are there universes with right-handed, left-handed or ambidextrous gods shepherding their chiral flocks? It's hard for us to conceive of life without amino acids, but to think it impossible is a human conceit. It's highly probable that we'll never know.

Scientists have puzzled over the origin of molecular handedness in living systems for decades. They argue heatedly over theories ranging from pure luck of the draw in primordial events to an unexplained bias in the fundamental forces of physics. Like the argument over the chicken and the egg, which came first, left handedness or life? Some thought that predominantly left-handedness must have come from outer space.[7] The discovery in 1970 that the Murchison meteorite contained amino acids, stimulated an increased interest in the possibility of an extraterrestrial origin of life. At the time, there was no evidence of other than a 50-50 mixture of optical isomers. Later studies by chemists **Jon R. Cronin** and **Sandra Pizzarello** at Arizona State University found a left-handed excess of 2 to 9%.[8] This leaves the questions of what could have caused a left-handed excess in outer space, for which several theories have been proposed, and whether life on other planets, if it exists or ever existed, will have primarily left or right amino acids or a *racemic* (50-50) mixture of the two contained in their proteins—or whatever it is that makes them tick.

German scientists made a discovery in 1994 that may be a clue to the dominance of lefties. While looking for ways to improve enantiomer yields, they found that when they applied a magnetic field, the raw materials reacted to produce primarily just one of the two mirror-image forms. A yield of 98% was obtained when they seeded the reaction solution with a small amount of the desired isomer. Organic chemist **Philip Kocienski** of the University of Southamptom in England speculated that the Earth's magnetic field might have had a similar effect during the evolution of organic molecules entering living systems at the origin of life. The

Germans' magnetic field was about 10,000 times stronger than the Earth's magnetic field. However, the relatively weak magnetic field of the Earth might have tilted the balance to the left during the presumed long period of time for the creation of life.[9]

While most synthetic production of chiral compounds usually results in equal amounts of the two mirror images, it is well-known that mirror-image isomers used in medicine often have very different biological effects. One form of the infamous thalidomide alleviates morning sickness, the other drastically affects fetal development. Many products pose similar problems. One form of limonene smells of oranges, the other of lemons. A potent carcinogen called benzo[*a*]pyrene, present in automobile exhaust, cigarette smoke, and barbecued meats, is attacked in the body by enzymes that form mirror-image breakdown products, both of which bind to DNA. But they align themselves in opposite directions; the right-handed isomer is carcinogenic, the other is not.[10]

Ibuprofen, the nonsteroidal anti-inflammatory drug contained in Motrin, Nuprin, and Advil, is a classic example of the difference in activity of two enantiomers. It is reported that one of the isomers of ibuprofen reaches therapeutic concentrations in the blood in 12 minutes compared to 30 minutes for the racemic mixture.[11] Only one, the (S)-enantiomer, is the active pain reliever. The (R)-isomer is ineffective, but is reported to be converted to the (S)-isomer in the body.[12] Studies indicated that one of the isomers of a marketed anti-asthmatic actually provoked constriction of the airways. A company in Japan introduced a chiral drug isomer for its specific action on the heart, but it was withdrawn from the market when it was found to have liver toxicity. An American company developed a beta-blocker for hypertension but found that the levo form is a vasodilator. Both forms alleviate hypertension by different mechanisms, suggesting that the racemate, i.e., both (+) and (-), might be better than either one alone. Another company developed a compound belonging to a class of calcium channel blockers that has potential to treat angina, hypertension, and asthma, and possibly glaucoma and impotence. The dextro-isomer turned out to have side effects, so the company turned to the levo form. When one company developed a drug intended as an antipsychotic by blocking the receptors for serotonin, they found that one of the enantiomers blocked serotonin and the other enhanced its effect.[13]

Pharmaceutical companies are vigorously pursuing enantiomers of chiral drugs for potential financial advantages: reduced dosage, greater effectiveness, reduced side effects, lower cost, or higher profits. One possibility is to develop right-handed antibiotics that would resist breakdown by the left-handed enzymes of bacteria. But the research required, so-called "bridging studies," is costly. It requires comparing what is already known about the product with what is unknown about the isomer under study. How much of the effectiveness is due to the isomer to be discarded? It may actually have some useful effect or it may modify the effect of the other isomer.[14] The Jekyll-Hyde qualities of chiral drugs pose a troubling dilemma, either for establishing safe doses or because of dangerous side effects.

CHAPTER 20

FDA: THE 300-YEAR WAR WITH POISONERS AND POLLUTERS

An early version of food and drug law in the United States was enactment of the Federal Food and Drug Act of 1906, administered by the Department of Agriculture. The Chief Chemist of the department was **Harvey W. Wiley** (1844-1930) who had campaigned against dishonest practices in food and drug packaging, and fought for a pure food and drug law. From the time the act was under consideration it was called "Wiley's bill". Wiley was born in Kent, Indiana. After graduating from Hanover College and the medical school in Indiana he became professor of chemistry at Purdue University. And from there, in 1907, to chief chemist in the Department of Agriculture, the first head of the government agency that evolved into what is now known as the U.S. Food and Drug Administration (FDA).[1] Wiley, at the age of 23, said in his commencement address at Hanover, "We are to carefully preserve that life which the author of nature has given us, for it was no idle gift." The FDA Papers, a periodical first published in 1967, carried in its masthead a picture of Dr. Harvey W. Wiley.[2]

The Food and Drug law of 1906 was modified and expanded by passage of the Food, Drug, and Cosmetics Act of 1938, at which time enforcement was moved from Agriculture to the Food and Drug Administration under the Department of Health, Education, and Welfare. The act was to assure the quality and purity of drugs by requiring accurate labeling of all medicinals, and to monitor contaminants of foods. Also enacted in 1906 was the Federal Meat Inspection Act, expanded later under the Poultry Products Inspection Act of 1957. These remained under supervision of the

Department of Agriculture because examination of sick animals required the knowledge of veterinarians. A Drug Amendments Act of 1962 was to establish the efficacy, as well as the safety, of new drugs because many of the new drugs under review were no better or even worse than established drugs of known quality. It was also the responsibility of the FDA to evaluate the toxicity of drugs already in use and if the toxicity was out of proportion to their therapeutic value, remove them from the market.

The Comprehensive Drug Abuse Prevention and Control Act of 1970 gave the Bureau of Narcotics and Dangerous Drugs under the Department of Justice the power to regulate the distribution of drugs that are apt to be abused.[3] The 1970 Act placed marijuana in schedule I (drugs with a high abuse potential and "*no* currently accepted medical use in treatment in the United States"). Despite the federal restriction, public production and use of marijuana became a multibillion dollar per year industry. A patchwork of state laws defying enforcement of the federal law permitted production, possession, and use of small amounts of marijuana, but the U.S. attorney general insisted that he would continue to prosecute violators of federal law. Use and control of marijuana is controversial. The ultimate outcome is yet to be determined.

Much of the pressure on Congress to do something about the unreliable quality of food and drug products came from the writing of **Upton Beale Sinclair** (1878-1968), much of whose work was exposing evils in various industries. *The Jungle* (1906), a fictionalized account of the unsanitary conditions and impurities in the Chicago meat processing industry, aroused such public anger and disgust that officials were prompted to investigate. The 1906 laws soon followed. Sinclair had been engaged by the socialist weekly newspaper *Appeal to Reason* with the intention of arousing sympathy for the overworked and poorly paid immigrant and minority workers in the stockyards. Sinclair said, "I aimed at the public's heart and by accident hit it in the stomach."

Upton Sinclair was born in Baltimore, Maryland. He attended The City College in New York and Columbia University. Notoriety from his writing led him to believe he could accomplish reforms if engaged in politics, so he ran for public office as a socialist but without success. He ran for governor of California on the Democrat ticket in 1934 but lost.

Even before the 1906 federal crackdown on food and drug abuses, there were many attempts to control dishonest, unsanitary, and dangerous practices. During colonial days people themselves, almost all without reliable refrigeration, had to be alert to the quality of food. It was prudent to smell food of all kinds, especially meat and fish. They examined flour for the presence of beetles or insect larvae. They checked fruit for mildew and for maggots. They cut open apples and pears looking for "worms," actually moth larvae. Bakers had an array of tricks to lower the cost of making bread, such as mixing clay or other contaminates with the dough. People took the purity of bread, "the staff of life," seriously. As early as 1646 a law was enacted by the General Court of Massachusetts Bay Colony that read: "It is ordered by the Court and Authority thereof...." There followed a detailed description of the kinds of bread sold, weights and prices, as well as who was authorized to enter suspect houses, and penalties. Laws in both England and the colonies prohibited adulteration of bread with ground up beans or chalk. The Massachusetts bread law was amended in 1652 because of "much deceit used by some bakers and others...." It required bakers to make all their bread in the legally required sizes. Massachusetts appointed a fish inspector in 1668 and in the same year passed a food additives law banning a kind of salt that had trash in it.

Massachusetts appears to have been the first of the colonies to inspect food exports. The Massachusetts General Court passed a law in 1641 that regulated the size of casks and required each town to select a packer to check containers of fish, beef, and pork, and determine that they were well seasoned (salted). The General Assembly of New York in 1773 prohibited bakers from selling bread unless made from flour that had passed an inspection required for exported flour. The law said that a consumer could sue the baker and get punitive damages of four shillings, plus costs, for each violation. An Act generally considered to be the first comprehensive food adulteration law in the United States was passed by the General Court of Massachusetts on March 8, 1785. Called the "Act against selling unwholesome Provisions", it set criminal penalties for violations.

An epidemic of poisoning in England in 1900 killed 6,000 people. Medical authorities were baffled, but soon traced the problem to beer. At first it was thought that lead was picked up from the pipes that carried beer from the barrels to the spigots. But investigators decided that the offending poison was arsenic derived from the processing of brewer's starch with acid contaminated with arsenic. A Royal Commission on Arsenical Poisoning went into action and in 1903 set a limit on the amount of arsenic permitted in drinks and foods. The maximum amount agreed on was 1.43 parts per million. This was called the "tolerance," an amount equal to about an aspirin tablet in a barrel of beer.

For many years the British did not seem to be greatly concerned about contamination of food until by 1925 large shipments of apples were being imported from the northwestern United States. Apple and pear growers, especially in Washington and Oregon, in order to produce marketable fruit were forced to spray their trees with an insecticide to control the coddling moth, *Carpocapsa pomonella*, the larvae of which are the "worms" in wormy apples and pears. The most effective insecticide was lead arsenate, which as the name implies is a combination of two powerful poisons, lead and arsenic. What tipped off the British was that the American fruit growers often had to spray repeatedly during the season, leaving a noticeably white coat of the poison on the fruit. British scientists found as much as ten times the tolerance for arsenic. The lingering British memory of their agonizing experience of arsenic in their ritual beer a quarter of a century earlier touched off a news media tirade on the danger of eating American apples. Authorities placed an embargo on American apples, refusing to allow importation unless the American growers could meet the tolerance for arsenic set by the Royal Commission.

A similar dispute occurred in America in 1919 when the Boston Health Department found that imported northwest pears contained the equivalent of a medicinal dose of arsenic on each pear. The city fathers promptly placed an embargo on western pears. The U.S. Bureau of Chemistry initiated a study of spray residues on fruit and vegetables. The Federal Food and Drug Act empowered the Bureau to establish safe standards and to confiscate contaminated food. Many shipments were held and shippers were ordered to remove visible residues. Chemical tests were not required, presumably due to limited money and manpower as well as the fact that methods for quick analysis of poisonous materials such as arsenic and lead had not been developed.

Again in 1925, the United States Bureau of Chemistry launched a campaign to seize and confiscate fruit that was overladen with poison. In one seizure of apples, the owner contested the action in federal court. Expert medical witnesses unanimously testified that the massive quantities of poison found were harmful to health. The decision in favor of the Bureau of Chemistry was a step in convincing farmers, packers, and shippers that killing insects with massive amounts of poison was only part of the problem. Most of the poison residue on the fruit would have to be removed. An effective procedure involved an acid wash and an alkaline wash with temperatures carefully controlled to avoid damaging the tender fresh fruit.

It's surprising that despite the numerous food laws of the colonies, statutes offering protection against ineffective drugs were absent. It was a time of frightening epidemics. Yellow fever, typhoid, scarlet fever, diphtheria, and measles were a way of life and death. Other diseases, dysentery, pneumonia, and tuberculosis, were as devastating but were endemic and taken as inevitable. Scurvy was prevalent in the colonies until it became common knowledge that **James Lind** (1716-1794), a Scottish Naval surgeon, had discovered in 1747 that lime juice would cure and prevent it. By 1774 the British navy made lime juice part of the daily rations for the "Limeys." Lind may have taken a cue from the Dutch who since 1593 had their naval ships carry sauerkraut for scurvy prevention.

Smallpox is said to have taken more colonist lives than all the British bullets. In addition to quarantines, hit-or-miss efforts to prevent the dreaded disease depended on "inoculation," application to a scratch in the skin with fluid from pustules of patients who hopefully were infected with a mild strain of the disease. Inoculation was a procedure introduced from Turkey to England and from there to America. Risky and controversial, the procedure was vigorously, sometimes violently, rejected by medical practitioners and the public, and just as vigorously promoted by **Cotton Mather** (1663-1728), an influential pastor of Boston's North Church. **Benjamin Franklin** (1706-1790), whose son died of smallpox, also supported the procedure as did **George Washington** (1732-1799) and **Thomas Jefferson** (1743-1826). By July 1776 the procedure was generally accepted in the colonies. A celebration in Boston was marked by mass inoculation of both troops and civilians ordered by the legislature on July 3. It was not until 1796 that a better and safer method of smallpox immunization was developed by **Edward Jenner** (1749-1823), an English country physician, initially by using fluid from comparatively benign cowpox pustules, and refined by others, especially **Louis Pasteur** (1822-1895).

FAST TRACK DRUG TESTS

In the early 1990s the FDA was criticized by both the public and pharmaceutical manufacturers for taking too long to approve new drugs. There was anxiety about the lack of effective drugs for treatment of AIDS. Heavy pressure was put on the FDA by private advocacy groups, industry, and Congress to streamline the way it did its job and to speed up approval of tests for new AIDS drugs. By 1992, FDA was persuaded to put all new drugs on fast track approval in which Congress gave the FDA authority to charge pharmaceutical companies "user fees" for the cost of faster drug testing.[4]

AIDS drugs and lucky patients were early beneficiaries of accelerated approval under the fast track policy. All new drugs were approved for marketing much sooner in the testing process than in the past. It eliminated months of testing, much to the satisfaction of pharmaceutical companies and Congress. But there was a backlash of an upsurge in failures and demands for recalls. The fast track system was criticized as making it possible for the pharmaceutical companies to market drugs before testing thoroughly enough to determine effectiveness and safety, endangering patients and possibly causing deaths. Fast track medications could be sold without restrictions or warnings.[5] The staff of Representative **Edward J. Markey** of Massachusetts, a senior member of the Energy and Commerce Committee that oversees the pharmaceutical industry, reported that by mid-2005 drug companies had completed only about half of the post-market clinical studies that they pledged to conduct for accelerated approval in 1992. The panel found that, of 91 studies committed, 21 had not even been started. **Thomas Fleming**, chairman of the biostatistics department at the University of Washington, who had served on FDA advisory committees, was quoted, "When accelerated approval has been provided, there is a loss of urgency."[6]

There was an increase in both dangerous drugs and delays in recalls, prompting **Sidney M. Wolfe**, M.D., director of Public Citizen's Health Research Group and editor of Public Citizen to publish a monthly report entitled *Worst Pills, Best Pills News* in which he warns consumers about the side effects of dangerous drugs, in some cases with the flat-out recommendation "do NOT use." According to Wolfe, 100,000 people die each year from adverse drug reactions of marketed drugs, and another 2,000,000 are seriously injured, with 1.5 million of those requiring hospitalization. He says that one in five new drugs have a significant safety problem after being approved.[7]

CHAPTER 21

A CHINESE PUZZLE

President Richard M. Nixon's (1913-1994) landmark state visit to the People's Republic of China in February, 1992, warmed the frosty relations with the Communist leaders in a way that gave promise of stimulating trade. Enthusiasm for globalization and the eagerness of industrialists to reduce costs by outsourcing production to countries with cheap labor, escalated imports to a flood of food and drug products beyond any possibility of the FDA monitoring more than a small fraction, probably less than 1%, for quality. According to **Caroline Smith De Waal**, food safety director at the Center for Science in the Public Interest in Washington D.C., China is the sixth leading supplier of Agricultural products to the U.S., and the third largest supplier of imported food generally including seafood. A result was that both the United States and China experienced problems with intentionally contaminated food and drugs made in China.

An adulterated food scandal occurred in 2007 when at least 1,000 cats and dogs in the U.S. died and thousands became sick after eating pet food traced to contaminates in wheat gluten imported from China as a pet food additive. The product contained two contaminates: melamine and cyanuric acid. Melamine is a high-nitrogen chemical that when added to food increases the nitrogen content, thus by the usual quick test, artificially inflates the apparent protein content. Cyanuric acid, also a high-nitrogen chemical, accomplishes the same nefarious purpose. Melamine is used in industry by reacting it with formaldehyde to make plastics or resins. Cyanuric acid is used in swimming pools and hot tubs to retard the breakdown of chlorine-based disinfectants.[1] **Birgit Puschner** and colleagues at the University of California at Davis found that melamine in combination with cyanuric acid caused kidney failure and death in cats.

They theorized that melamine and cyanuric acid when ingested react to form insoluble crystals in the kidneys.²

Chinese officials said they had shut down two factories that had produced the deadly pet food ingredients. They also closed down a plant that supplied a product mistakenly labeled "glycerin" intended for use in a cough syrup in Panama. The product was actually diethylene glycol, a toxic chemical used as an automobile antifreeze. Panama's Social Security Agency made 450 bottles of the syrup for distribution to the poor. There were 67 confirmed deaths.³

Melamine also figured in a disastrous contamination of milk produced in China and sold to Chinese citizens. The milk was deliberately contaminated with melamine. As with pet food, when the high-nitrogen chemical is added to diluted milk, it artificially inflates the apparent protein content. The contaminated milk sickened 53,000 babies and caused thousands of Chinese babies to develop kidney stones. At least four died from the ailment. One baby formula contained 2563 mc/kg of melamine which added 1% apparent crude protein. To stem public anger the court in Shijiazhuang put 21 defendants on trial. **Tian Wenhua**, 66, was chairwoman of the manufacturer of contaminated baby formula that sickened about 300,000 babies of which six died. She received a life sentence. **Zhang Yujun**, 40, a former dairy farmer, was accused of endangering public security by selling 600 tons of melamine powder, sold as "protein powder." He and **Geng Jinping**, 48, convicted of selling poisonous food, were executed July 16, 2007. Defendant, **Zhang Yanzhang**, was sentenced to life in prison. Another man got a suspended death sentence which in China usually means life in prison.⁴

Execution seemed to be the Chinese way of quickly putting a stop to contaminating food or drugs. Five executives of a drug manufacturer were put on trial for making a faulty injectable drug that killed 13 people. They were accused of negligently using diethyleneglycol instead of the benign but more expensive propyleneglycol. The cheaper diethyleneglycol had been approved by China's State Food and Drug Administration (SFDA). The former head of SFDA, **Zheng Xiaoyu**, 62, was accused of accepting $850,000 in bribes in exchange for approving drugs. He was executed July 16, 2007.⁵

On July 17, 2007 the U.S. House Energy & Commerce Subcommittee on Oversight & Investigations, chaired by representative **Bart Stupak** (D-

Mich.) said that the recent food safety incidents raised questions about the FDA's ability and authority to regulate food and drug imports. There was concern about some of the products from China—contaminated seafood, toothpaste containing ethyleneglycol, and the poisonous melamine in wheat gluten imported for adding to domestically produced pet food. Stupak pointed out that FDA inspects less than 1% of food imports and takes samples from only a small fraction of that. He criticized FDA's plan to close seven of 13 laboratories that test both domestic and imported food. **David Nelson**, an investigator on the oversight subcommittee, said that the FDA has no authority to visit foreign process plants for fish and other produce. It allows imports at more than 300 U.S. ports but has inspectors at only 90 of them.[6]

Contamination of the blockbuster drug, heparin, that was blamed for up to 81 deaths and 785 severe allergic reactions, prompted the FDA to send warning letters to two Chinese suppliers citing failure to follow drug manufacturing practice. Baxter International, with about half of the U.S. market, began recalling the drug in January, 2008, in the belief that it was intentionally contaminated. Scientific Protein Laboratories, a U.S. company, owned a majority stake in the Chinese company that made the active ingredient in Baxter's heparin.[6]

Heparin is an anticoagulant, commonly given to patients undergoing heart surgery or kidney dialysis. Administration must be carefully controlled because overdose causes bleeding. FDA identified the contaminant as oversulfated chondroitin sulfate. They also found in some lots a recognized heparin impurity not known to be harmful. The importance of Baxter's heparin is indicated by another blockbuster anticoagulant called Lovenox, made by France's Sanofi-Aventis. Lovenox was rated the 15th best selling drug in the world with 2009 sales of $4.5 billion.[7, 8, 9]

The Grocery Manufacturers/Food Products Association (GMA) in 2007 recommended, among other things, that the FDA budget be increased so more scientists and inspectors could be hired. The number of contaminated products imported from China eventually led the FDA to establish its own personnel and stations in China to monitor the safety of drug and manufactured food products intended for shipment to the U.S. In February 2008, FDA announced that it was sending a team of inspectors to China. The team would include a chemist who speaks Chinese fluently and an expert in drug manufacturing technology. By early 2008, **Murray M.**

Lumpkin, FDA's deputy commissioner for international and special programs reported that they had placed staffs at the U.S. embassy in Beijing and at the U.S. consulates in Shanghai and Guangzhou.[10]

CHAPTER 22

A BLOODY SHAME

A sad episode in the history of healing was the centuries following the stagnating influence of Galen on the medical establishment during which patients were subjected to a staggering array of treatments that were useless or worse. The most deadly because it led the pack as the favorite lead-off treatment for any disease, or simply to purify the system, was the practice of bleeding, often called blood-letting.

Medical historian **Howard Haggard** speculated that bleeding originated with primitive people "as a sort of peace offering to the ghosts and spirits. A man gave some of his blood to flatter them into favoring him…a human sacrifice to appease the gods."[1] The Greek philosopher **Empedocles** (about 492-432 B.C.) came up with the idea of four basic elements of the universe (*water*, *air*, *fire*, and *earth*). It became clear to physicians of the school of **Hippocrates** that diseases were not caused by the arrows of Apollo, the fury of the gods, or demons but by disruptions of elements in the human body. The troublesome elements eventually were called the four humors: *black bile*, *yellow bile*, *phlegm*, *and blood*. The logical and most responsive of the four humors to deal with was blood, the most abundant fluid of the body, the most accessible, and for safety required the services of someone equipped for surgery. From the time of Hippocrates, who said that he "avoided surgery, leaving it to those who do that sort of thing," professional healers, despised surgery as beneath their calling.

But the popular idea that ailments and diseases were caused by unclean things in the blood led to the reasoning that disease could best be dealt with by removing the "bad blood." Barbers seized the opportunity to be helpful. Known as *barber-surgeons*, they became a recognized profession. The barber pole colored in spiraling red and white, red for the blood and white for the bandage, survives today as a sign of a barber shop, centuries after its invention. The barber surgeons thrived on the conviction of patients and non-patients alike that bleeding was good for them. Even furriers, cobblers and tinkers managed to get in on the act. An early barber surgeon was a shadowy figure named **Gilbert** (1180-1250) who roamed Europe and did a bit of writing. He was known as **Gilbertus Anglicus** because he claimed that he was born in England. He believed in drawing blood for the relief of pain.

Barber surgeons, though despised as lowly exploiters, gained some notoriety in 1540 when **King Henry VIII** (ruled 1509-1546) was called upon to deal with a quarrel between the apothecaries and the barber surgeons.[2] A barber surgeon who gained recognition and status was **Ambroise Pare'** (1510-1590), called "the father of modern surgery." He was born in Boug Hersent, France, where he became the village barber, taking on whatever surgery was asked for. He obtained useful experience by serving in the army as a barber surgeon, and during peaceful intervals served as surgeon to kings **Henry II, Francis II, Charles IX, and Henry III**, and engaged in extensive writing. He was the first prominent healer to criticize popular but useless remedies and practices, and to propose changes. As for blood-letting, he pointed out that when nature was trying to heal, and every ounce of blood was needed, "bleeding weakened the patient beyond all hope of recovery."[3] Other practitioners ridiculed and denounced Pare' for using ligatures instead of a red-hot iron to stop bleeding and the common use of boiling oil as a surgical dressing.

A law passed in Massachusetts in 1649, and later in New York in 1684, entitled An Act Respecting Chirurgions, Midwives and Physicians, said that "practitioners were to adhere to known approved rules of the art" unless they consulted qualified persons and obtained patient consent. There was no provision for enforcement. The state of the art for healing in colonial times is seen in the medical treatment of President **George Washington** in his last illness, probably a streptococcus infection. On December 12, 1799, he took his daily horseback ride around Mount Vernon. The day was cold, with snow turning to sleet and rain. After about five hours he returned and sat down for dinner without changing his damp clothes. The next day he woke up with a sore throat and went for a walk. That night (Dec. 14) he awakened Martha about 2 or 3 A.M. He could hardly speak and felt very sick but would not let her send for a doctor until dawn. His long-time friend and doctor, **James Craik**, rushed to Mount Vernon as soon as called. Washington had already called in an overseer to drain about a cup of blood from his veins. Dr. Craik bled him again and two more doctors arrived in the afternoon. The treatment given Washington is described in detail by FDA reporter **Wallace F. Janssen**:[4] Washington was given a mixture of molasses, vinegar, and butter, which he was unable to swallow. He was forced to eat sal volatile (a menthol salve), he was bled a pint, his throat was wrapped in flannel soaked in sal volatile, his feet were bathed in warm water, a blister (poultice) of Spanish flies (cantharides) was applied to his throat, he was bled another pint, made to gargle with sage tea and vinegar, then bled again. As he worsened he was bled a full quart and given a laxative of calomel (a compound of mercury and chlorine) and an emetic of tartar (calcium or potassium phosphate). One of the physicians, a young man, suggested the new procedure called tracheotomy (surgically opening the windpipe below the point of mucous obstruction, so the patient can breathe). He was overruled by the older physicians and instead, plasters of wheat bran were applied to his feet. Soon afterward George Washington died, December 14, 1799, at the age of 67.

Blister of Spanish fly refers to the medical use of the secretion from "blister beetles", *Cantharis vesicatoria*, also known as Spanish fly. The juice, called cantherides, from the Greek *kantharis* for "beetle," contains the active ingredient *cantharidin* which is a vesicant, that is, causes a blister when in contact with the skin. The extracted juice or pulverized dried beetles was used with wine as a powerful aphrodisiac by indulgent citizens of Rome. But cantharidin is such a strong irritant that it causes inflammation of the kidneys and reproductive system. Many of the revelers must have had their health impaired or died from the poison. Gladiators, who used the powdered beetles routinely followed up with hot baths to remove the toxin by the sweat glands. **Ibn Wahshiyya**, an Arabian toxicologist who practiced in the ninth century AD, wrote about poisons and their antidotes. He described the preparation of blister beetles for assassinations, a political weapon commonly used in medieval times. One thousandth of an ounce (about 0.5 mg per kg of body weight) would be lethal to the average size person.

By all accounts the General had rugged strength and vitality. It took a lot of "healing" to kill the Father of the country. But without antibiotics he could have died of the illness anyway.

Roll the screen back about a century to February 2, 1685. King **Charles II** of England (ruled 1660-1685) was being shaved in his bedroom when he fell from his chair in convulsions and unconscious. Possibly from a stroke or embolism. He opened his eyes once or twice and remained alive for several days. His physician, one of a dozen or more assembled to treat the king, was ready to start the bleeding, purging, enemas, and an astounding array of medicines: There were 2 bleedings at start, and more bleeding of unspecified number later. Medicines that could not be swallowed were forced down the dying king's throat.[5, 6]

By comparison, George Washington's last days a century later were benign and peaceful.

When yellow fever hit Philadelphia in 1792, killing more than 3,000 people, many fled in panic. Most of those who remained held a cloth saturated with garlic juice to their noses or smeared their clothing with tar, or both. **Dr. Benjamin Rush** (1745-1813) bled all of the yellow fever patients who would submit to it.[5] Blood-letting was popular as the standard first-line treatment for almost all diseases in the fifteenth, sixteenth, and seventeenth centuries, and remained a choice of some physicians as late as the eighteenth and early nineteenth centuries. Medical historian Howard Haggard told how **Guy Patin**, a prominent Paris physician of the seventeenth century, bled himself seven times for a head cold, and bled his son twenty times within a few days for an illness.[6]

Bleeding was by no means the only popular treatment. In later years purging often took its place as the first step in treatment, often by an apothecary without a doctor's order. Purgatives were usually the powerful salt of antimony or calomel (a salt of mercury). Enemas were another commonly overused treatment, also a profitable business for the apothecary, often performed by his assistant. The enema became so popular that barbers sometimes took the business.[7]

Drugs consisted largely of herbals, most of which had no recognizable value except to satisfy the idea of "the more the better." Physicians and pharmacists were inclined to toss dozens of herbals into the mix. The inclusion of filthy or poisonous ingredients popular in ancient Egypt were abandoned in favor of mostly harmless substances. (Snake poisons were popular in Egypt. The story is told that Cleopatra tested the poison of the asp on her slaves before applying it to herself. A drug called theriac was a popular remedy. It contained 37 to 63 ingredients composed of the flesh of vipers. It later became known as treacle.)[8]

Despite the wisdom of Pare's observation that blood is needed when one is sick, most people continued to believe that bad blood was the main source of trouble. When physicians first began to consider the value of transfusions they wondered if blood from another person would change the temperament of the person receiving it. They even wondered if transfusing sheep's blood to a dog would transform the animal to a sheep. One physician suggested curing marital problems between husband and wife with mutual transfusions from one to the other, thus, by sharing the same traits they would enjoy the same interests in a compatible life. It was not until the seventeenth century that crude attempts were made to take blood from the vein of one person and transfer it to the vein of another.[9, 10]

PART V
HEALTHFUL LIVING

23 S̲anitation

24 T̲he S̲olution

25 T̲he W̲ater W̲ar

26 F̲eeders A̲nd B̲reeders

CHAPTER 23

SANITATION

The glamour of wonder drugs and magic bullets in the cure of diseases need not divert our attention from the basic need that is prevention, and that the first step in prevention of many diseases is cleanliness. During the Ice Age 15,000 years ago there may have been no more than 100,000 people on earth. Disposal of waste was no problem. Wild animals consumed discarded bones and scraps, and human waste was taken care of by a quick visit to the woods. The answer was the dilution of a small amount of detritus in an expansive environment.

The phenomenal reproductive capacity of *Homo sapiens* changed things. Relatives clung together in food gathering, and clans cooperated for protection. The invention of agriculture brought them together in villages, and specialization of industries led to cities of larger and larger size, culminating in evermore dense congestion with increasing accumulation of wastes and exposure to diseases. Humans are not the tidiest of animals, as any cat admirer knows. But it must be said that early human cultures developed innovative sanitation practices sadly forgotten during the rapid growth of human activity during the Middle Ages and the Industrial Revolution. Maybe people were too busy getting rich to think about the seriousness of their inattention to the accumulation of human waste, much as today we prefer to ignore global warming because to do anything serious about it would be "bad for business."

The first people known to become adept at sanitation were the Harappan of the Indus Valley, about 2500 BC. They built household water supplies, bathing facilities, and drainage systems. Bathrooms had waterproof floors, and latrines with seats were built into some houses. There were sloping channels built through walls that emptied into either pottery receptacles or outside drains. At Mohenjo-Daro the houses had drains that emptied into a sewer system under the street leading to a central cesspool. Brick manhole covers allowed for repairs and cleaning. Citizens of the ancient Indus would have been aghast at the chaotic sanitation practices in some parts of the modern world with sewage sluiced along roadside gutters into open sewers where the vagaries of wind, vermin, and bacteria make them not only aesthetically offensive but a constant threat to human health and welfare.

Akhetaton, an Egyptian city built during the XVIII Dynasty (1580-1340 BC) had upper-class houses equipped with bathrooms, drains, braziers, and stands for holding vessels of drinking and washing water. In Crete about 2000 BC the palaces had running water brought in through tile pipes with finely fitted joints, and latrines with running water. Similar advances in hygiene were made by the early Greeks but it remained for the engineering genius of the Romans to make the greatest achievements of the ancient world in sanitation and waste disposal.

Nearly every house in Rome had a cistern, water faucets, and pipes of lead or terra cotta. Excavations at Pompeii reveal a central distributing system that brought water to each house. Public sit-down latrines with running water can be seen in the ruins of the Greek and Roman seaport city of Ephesus (now in Turkey). Private toilets with running water, such as those at the villa of Emperor **Hadrian** (117-138) near Rome, were a common luxury.

One of the aspects of Venus was **Venus Cloacina**, the goddess of drains. The *cloacae* of ancient Rome were laid out to drain the marshy grounds between the hilly areas of the city. The Cloaca Maxima, dating from about the sixth century BC, drained the Forum and discharged into the Tiber. Today it would be called a "combined sewer" because it received both sewage and surface drainage water. The Cloaca Maxima was so well constructed that it still serves the city. It is 10½ feet wide, 14 feet high, arched in stone, and paved with lava in polygonal blocks. Cities in the provinces also had drainage systems, flush latrines, and sewage storage pits. Public latrines as they appeared 1500 years ago can still be seen in cities in northern Africa.

Two of the most important discoveries in sanitation were the invention of toilet paper and the water closet. The first appeared when papyrus was still used only for recording and communicating knowledge. The water closet was devised by the people of the Indus Valley 4000 years before it was reinvented in 1596 by the Englishman **Sir John Harington** (1561-1612), godson of **Queen Elizabeth I** (1533-1603). Harington described his invention in a publication entitled *A New Discourse on a State subject, Called the Metamorphosis of Ajax* printed in London in 1596. ("Jacks" was slang for privy.[1]) The Queen is said to have had it installed at Richmond Palace. Harington's device was modified and perfected by **Thomas Crapper**, a British manufacturer of sanitation equipment. Three manhole covers in the cloisters of Westminster Abbey bear the name of T. Crapper & Co. Ltd., Sanitary Engineers. Crapper is credited with developing the water closet in essentially its modern form and being the first to make it widely available. According to Christopher Hamlin writing in the *American Scientist*, "It is widely agreed that many more people lack adequate sanitation than lack water. The usual figure for the former is 2.6 billion people. According to Black and Fawcett, if the flush toilet is the standard that must be met for sanitation to be considered adequate, the number of people lacking it rises to 4 billion."[2]

Except for development of the "crapper," and its eventual acceptance during the nineteenth century, there were few advances in hygiene since the forgotten innovations of the ancient world. Even the finest palaces had nothing more than open privies. The congestion of people in cities made living conditions grim. Typical in all big cities were the tenements of Glasgow where there were no drains, or even privies. Human waste was left lying in the courtyards next to houses. In other towns there were no private lavatories and only two or three public privies in the better sections of the city. Things were no better in other European cities and in some it was worse. It was the practice of citizens of Paris to use chamber pots for excreta, and when they were filled, to empty the contents out the window and into the street below with a warning shout for anyone nimble enough to benefit from it. A minor innovation by Paris householders was the use of cesspits periodically emptied into wagons to carry it away, or emptied in the middle of the night into the gutters of the streets. Historian **David Barnes** wrote of the "Great Stink of Paris" of the summer of 1880 and another smell episode fifteen years later. The mass execution of communists after the defeat by Germany in 1870-1871 during which at least 20,000 people were summarily shot had left Paris with a shortage of artisans and plumbers. It was not until about 1903 that houses in Paris with sewer connections began to outnumber those with cesspits. At the beginning of World War I the city still had more than 25,000 cesspits.

Early London had a makeshift sewage system for part of its population of nearly 3 million people. The effluent was collected in a single huge cesspit in the center of the city. During the hot summer months the stench was nearly beyond human endurance. Thousands of backyard cesspools frequently overflowed into the streets.

Several episodes of so-called Asiatic cholera struck London as well as other parts of the world in the early to mid-nineteenth century. An epidemic of cholera apparently originated in India in 1817 from where a pandemic spread throughout Southeast Asia, East Africa, the Middle East, and the Caucasus. A second cholera pandemic, also originating in India, raged for eleven years from 1826 to 1837 during which it also spread to Europe, reaching America in 1832. An epidemic of the disease struck England and Wales, especially hitting London in 1831-1833 during which 20,000 people died of the disease. Cholera struck England and Wales again in 1848-1849 during which 50,000 died, then again in 1954 killing 30,000 victims in London.

Cholera (a name derived from the Greek *choler* for yellow bile) is a dreadful disease, an infection of the small intestine caused by the bacterium *Vibrio cholerae*, spread by ingesting water or food contaminated with excrement of infected people, though the causative organism would not be known until three decades after the 1854 London epidemic. The bacteria produce a toxin that induces the intestine to secrete enormous amounts of watery fluid along with salts and minerals. Symptoms begin 1 to 3 days after infection. They usually start with sudden, painless, watery diarrhea and watery vomit, sometimes causing a loss in fluid of more than 1 quart an hour, but usually less. In severe cases, the loss of water and depletion of salts leads to severe dehydration with agonizing thirst, muscle cramps, and weakness. Unless treated, the reduced blood volume and increased concentration of salts can lead to kidney failure, shock, and coma. If untreated, more than 50 percent of the victims die. Treatment not known then but now known to be highly effective can reduce the loss to 1 percent. Rapid replacement of lost fluids, salts, and minerals and early treatment with tetracycline or another antibiotic usually stops the diarrhea in 48 hours.[3]

By the time of the London epidemic of 1854 the city had made dubious progress in sanitation. Sewage was deposited in the Thames River although there was still a scattering of privies or worse, and private and public wells. Thousands of Crapper's water closets had been installed, adding an insufferable burden to an already reeking river. During what a newspaper called "The Great Stench" during the summer of 1858, politicians fled the House of Parliament on the river's embankment although some attended sessions with handkerchiefs held to their noses.

Several water companies took water from the Thames and piped it to various parts of the city. Two of the companies took their water from the tidal area below the sewage outfall. In one case water from below the outfall was piped along a street parallel to another line with water from above the outfall so that some houses along the street received clean water and others received a fecal cocktail resulting in a puzzling distribution of cholera cases. Parliament ordered the companies to shift their intakes upstream but some were slow to do it.

A London physician, **John Snow** (1813-1858) had become intrigued with the spotty occurrence of cholera cases throughout the city and undertook a detailed study in an effort to find the cause and distribution of the epidemic. The son of a farmer, Snow was apprenticed to a surgeon at the age of fourteen and obtained his medical degree in 1844 from the University of London. When he heard of the use of ether as an anesthetic by the American dentist, **William Morton** (1819-1868), he studied ways of using it in surgery, published a book on his method and became the pre-eminent anesthetist in the country, selected to administer anesthetic to Queen Victoria at the first assisted royal birth. But his greater fame came from his epidemiology studies. A treatise, *On the Mode of Communication of Cholera*, published in 1855, described a study in which he concluded that cholera during the epidemics of 1828-1839 and 1853-1854 was spread by contaminated water. Snow cited 500 deaths occurring within 10 days. He had mapped areas of the city, pinpointing cholera cases and correlating them with the water supply, for example, deaths in households along the two parallel water lines, one clean, the other from the polluted tidal part of the Thames.

Snow's conclusion that cholera was spread by contaminated water was rejected and blithely ignored by London physicians and politicians who were thoroughly imbued with the *miasma*, i.e., vapor, theory of its spread, and the disease itself they believed to be an imbalance of the four humors: blood, phlegm, yellow bile, and black bile, following principles established and handed down for centuries. They countered Snow with the claim that contaminated water was being used long before cholera appeared. How could it be the cause of the epidemic? On the other hand, they said, poisons might be airborne in the London stench.

The finding for which Snow is most cited was the case of a polluted well. He lived near an area of London called Soho, a neglected area in which there had been an unusually large number of cholera cases. He noticed that nearly all of the people who used water from a shallow well on Broad Street had sickened with cholera. The well had a hand-operated pump and supplied water to about a two block area. Snow said the water had "an offensive smell." No wonder. The well was not only near a sewer line it was also a few feet from a leaking cesspool. At a nearby prison (workhouse) where conditions were cramped and filthy, there had been no cholera. It had its own well. Nor was there any at the nearby Lion Brewery which also had its own well. On September 7, 1854, Snow asked the Parish Board of Guardians to disable the pump at the polluted Soho well. They complied, probably more out of respect for the distinguished surgeon-anesthetist than acceptance of the idea that polluted water had caused the cholera. Sometime after the epidemics had subsided, the pump was reactivated. Snow could not protest. He died June 16, 1858.[4]

The city continued to improve the water supply. Withdrawal of water from the sewage-laden tidal area of the Thames was stopped, and all water was required to be taken from upstream sources. Fear of miasma from the stench prompted building a sewer system that deposited the sewage into the Thames below the city. It became fully operational in the mid-1870s, and still serves London.

Much has been written of John Snow's remarkable work by admirers who have anointed him as a hero for discovering that cholera is "communicated" by polluted water, and bringing the epidemic to an end. In fact, the epidemic had run much of its course by the time the Broad Street pump was disabled. But Snow was a hero in the sense that his thorough study of the cause and spread of a disease set the gold standard for epidemiology, augmented later by the emerging sciences of bacteriology, parasitology, and eventually the discovery of viruses. It's not clear how much influence he had on the medical and public health establishments dominated by the antiquated notion that diseases are caused by miasmas or other atmospheric causes or combinations. To be sure, they moved intakes of the water supply to cleaner sources, and their action of dumping the sewage down river relocated the stench. They made the right decisions apparently out of the innate human disgust of stench and its implication of filth.[5]

CHAPTER 24

THE SOLUTION

London's solution to the waste problem was *dilution*, with care to take its fresh river water supply above the pipe outlets that dumped sewage into the Thames. The UN Environment Program (UNEP) estimates that 2.6 billion people have no access to basic sanitation.[1] But, in advanced parts of the world, pipes and tunnels were built to carry raw sewage to the nearest river or body of water. In the United States, the Mississippi River typically became a giant repository for human and industrial waste along its more than two thousand meandering miles to the Gulf of Mexico. "Old Man River" and its tributaries is one of the largest river systems in the world, draining about one-third of the total area of the United States. What a temptation! Polluted neighbors typically pollute other neighbors. Chicago takes its drinking water from Lake Michigan and so that it does not dump its sewage back into the lake to pollute itself, instead sluices it into the Mississippi River through a man-made canal.

Trouble appeared in the Great Lakes as early as 1925 when fishermen suffered a collapse in the cisco fishery of Lake Erie, only the first in a series of pollution problems. What seemed like an almost limitless supply of fresh water for coastal cities and industries, was transformed by the irresistible convenience of such vast bodies of water for disposal of human and all manner of industrial waste. By 1938, the city of Green Bay had to close its bathing beaches for health reasons. The state of Illinois sued the city of Milwaukee for polluting Lake Michigan.

Molecules of water that travel down the rivers in densely populated areas are said to pass through human physiological systems several times before reaching the ocean. It is repellent to think of drinking in the afternoon, molecules that were flushed into the river by our upstream neighbors in the morning, added to the vast quantities of domestic and industrial waste already present. The twentieth century's increase in population centers and industrial activity demanded sewage cleanup, resulting in a mixed bag of methods. The most primitive sewage treatment was the outhouse, consisting of a small building either detached or attached, with a seat over a deep pit. Although first used in cities lacking sewage facilities, it was a common sight at farmhouses during the expansion of agriculture in the western United States. In more civilized areas it was replaced with a septic tank and indoor plumbing but most cities required connection to a sewer line designed to deposit the untreated waste in the most convenient waterway. In medium to large centers of population it soon became apparent that some form of treatment would be required for public health and sanitary reasons. The first step known as *primary treatment* consists of screening out solids and floating debris, removing grease and scum, running the sewage into so-called grit chambers to remove sand and solids that could damage pumps, then running the sewage directly into settling tanks where a *sludge* is formed consisting of 94 to 99 percent water. The sludge has to be disposed of, which in some cases is done by letting it dry in beds and removing the water by filtration. Because the sludge itself can be a pollution problem, a better method is to bring about microbial decomposition in so-called *digestion tanks* before drying. Various methods are used to get rid of the dewatered sludge such as hauling it away to a landfill or converting it to a fertilizer.

One of the greatest innovations of the twentieth century was the introduction of chemical treatment of drinking water to prevent waterborne diseases and epidemics caused by bacteria and viruses. Disinfection by chlorination is now an essential measure used by almost all municipal water systems. The strength of chlorine does not last long, so enough is added to the water for it to keep the pipes of the distribution system clear of pathogenic organisms, rarely causing detectable off-flavor compared to fresh well water. Chlorination requires monitoring, not for flavor, but for production of potentially harmful toxins caused by reactions with naturally occurring materials in the water. The most common by-products of chlorination are chloroform, sometimes referred to as trihalomethane, and related so-called haloacetic acids, allowable limits of which were set by the U.S. Environmental Protection Agency under the Safe Drinking Water Act. In January, 2002, a ruling lowered the annual maximum average of trihalomethanes (THMs), mainly chloroform, to 80 parts per billion from the previous 100 parts per billion set in a 1979 ruling. A wide range of potentially harmful substances unrelated to the use of chlorine, are monitored, including arsenic, barium, and uranium.

Another method of disinfecting water is with ozone, a highly active form of oxygen (O_3) that has been used for the purpose on a limited scale for over a hundred years. It is highly effective and avoids the undesirable byproducts of chlorination. Ozone destroys a wider range of pathogenic organisms than chlorination and removes disagreeable odors and tastes that may be present. The Metropolitan Water District of Southern California is spending $856 million on a retrofit program to convert all of its five treatment plants to ozone disinfection.

Fluoride has the distinction of being the only medicine routinely added to drinking water (medicine in that it adds a crucial element for strengthening the teeth and bones). Fluorides contain the element fluorine, which belongs to a group of chemicals that includes bromine, chlorine, iodine, and fluorine, collectively called the *halogens* from a Greek word meaning "salt producing." (They all form chemical combinations consisting of salts such as sodium chloride, the common table salt). Fluorine in its elemental state is, like chlorine, a gas. But in nature it is always found in various combinations of minerals. Fluorine in its various combinations makes up about 0.1 percent of the earth's crust. Plants take it up from the soil and water and animals derive it from food, water, and minerals. Thus, fluorides are part of the structure of teeth and bones of most vertebrate animals.

The amount of fluoride in natural water varies. If it's too low children's teeth do not develop normally and are prone to tooth decay, and if it's too high the teeth are faulty and develop an unsightly black discoloration. The effect of tooth decay from drinking water of certain districts was noted by **Vetruvius Pollio**, a great Roman architect and builder of the first century BC. He said the water at Susa, the ancient capital of Persia, was for that reason unfit for human consumption although the relationship to low fluoride content was unknown. Tooth impairment of a different nature called *denti neri* (black teeth) was noticed in later times among people in the vicinity of Vesuvius and other places in Italy where the soils of volcanic origin contain large amounts of fluorides.

The effects of excess fluoride were noted early in the twentieth century in the United States by **Dr. F. S. McKay**, a dentist who practiced in Colorado Springs where the water contained about 2 ppm (parts per million) fluoride. The condition was called "Colorado brown stain." Since then, other areas have been identified as having fluorine concentrations of 2 ppm or above and correlated with the prevalence of mottled teeth and abnormal bone structure. Fluoride as high as 10 to 14 ppm have been detected but that is unusual. (Soils average about 300 ppm). In some high concentration areas livestock are affected, some seriously enough to be incapacitated. Grass and grains grown in such areas take up quantities of fluorides. Cattle are the most susceptible of the farm animals but also affected are sheep, swine, horses, turkeys, and chickens in that order of decreasing susceptibility.

Fluoride has been added to drinking water supplies in the United States since 1945. Of the 50 largest cities, 43 fluoridate their water. Some states mandate that all water suppliers fluoridate the water to within the optimum level range, ordinarily set at 0.7 to 1.3 ppm, with a maximum allowable amount of 2 ppm. Because the intake of water is highly variable an effort is made to add only enough fluoride to meet a minimum level. In the southern parts of the United States the optimum is generally considered to be between 0.5 and 0.7 ppm. In some cities the amount is raised in the winter and lowered in the summer.

CHAPTER 25

THE WATER WAR

In many parts of the world a safe and abundant water supply is a luxury. And it is becoming increasingly scarce because of the demand. There is a link between safe water and public health. The UN Environment Program (UNEP) says that 1.1 billion people lack access to safe drinking water. It is apt to be critical in desert and semi-desert areas. Arid southern California is a classic example. By the early twentieth century it became apparent to the influential people of Los Angeles that if their dream of expansion and promising real estate development were to continue they would have to bring water in from an outside source. They found ten times what they were looking for, 240 miles north of the city in the fertile Owens Valley, a thriving agricultural area with an abundant supply of water, the runoff from the Sierra Nevada range, the magnificent beauty of which is augmented by the heavy winter snowpack that in the spring feeds numerous streams and lakes. The Owens River flowed from its headwaters in the Sierras southward east of Mt. Whitney (at 14,494 feet the highest in the 48 contiguous states) and continued to meander for 125 miles into Owens Lake. To get that water to Los Angeles took some scheming. How they did it is told by **Abraham Hoffman** in *Vision or Villainy*.[1]

The leading visionary or villain, depending on whether you're a Los Angeles booster or an Owens Valley settler, was **Frederick Eaton**, a civil engineer and former mayor of Los Angeles. Eaton was a native Californian, actually born in Los Angeles September 23, 1855. His father, a Harvard graduate, came to California to make his fortune during the gold rush. Failing that, he set up a law practice in Los Angeles. His son Fred's schooling ended at the age of thirteen when the superintendent, impressed with his talent for drawing, assigned him to teach other pupils the art. Still thirteen, he began an apprenticeship at the Los Angeles Water Company and within five years became superintendent. To compensate for his lack of formal education he applied himself diligently to a study of engineering and fifteen years after becoming superintendent he resigned to go into private practice as a civil engineer. A specialty of his was designing irrigation works for land owners. He was elected to the office of City Engineer of Los Angeles and became prominent in civic circles and social clubs. He won an election for the city's highest office and became mayor December 15, 1898.

After his term of office Eaton took his family on an extended vacation through the Owens Valley and the eastern Sierra, giving him an opportunity to study the water and power potentialities of the region. Upon his return to Los Angeles he visited his close friend, **William Mulholland** who had replaced him as superintendent of the water company, and described in glowing terms the possibility of a water source for the city. Mulholland was unimpressed. He said the city had plenty of water. But after a tour through the Owens Valley with Eaton, he became an enthusiastic promoter of the idea. They gained the support of important city officials who initiated plans to finance the project with bond issues.

Fred Eaton pitched in without delay. Returning to the Owens Valley in the guise of an investor wanting to buy cattle land, he quietly proceeded to acquire options in property along the Owens River including water rights. Negotiations were always friendly and unhurried. Ranchers saw him mostly as a bit gullible. When they resisted his offers, he readily met their demands. A big success was an option he negotiated on land owned by Thomas B. Rickey, a cattle rancher whose company owned 22,380 acres in Inyo and Mono counties. Eaton closed the deal on the land plus 4,000 head of cattle for $450,000, paying $100 for the option. Later Rickey said he didn't know of Eaton's intentions. Eaton was able to wrap up options on nearly all the property bordering about a hundred miles of the river. He had an agreement with the city for him to retain title in his name to several thousand acres. Eaton, the water company, and city officials had kept the negotiations a secret to avoid the prospect of speculators dipping in and demanding high prices. News reporters were cooperating but the *Los Angeles Times* spilled the beans in a news story on July 25, 1905. *The Examiner* was angry at being scooped and bragged about having kept the faith. Residents of the Owens Valley were outraged. It was the beginning of a dispute with the government and in court battles that lasted for over a hundred years.

A player in the game to get federal approval for transferring water from one watershed to another was **Joseph Lippincott**, a civil engineer employed in the Hydrographic Service of the U.S. Geological Survey as supervisor of the Service's activity in California. He had an understanding, not unusual in some branches of service, that he could engage in private practice on the side. On June 17, 1902, the U.S. Congress had passed the *National Reclamation Act* intended to assist irrigation projects in the arid west. Lippincott, whose home was in Los Angeles, was accused of having a conflict of interest. He was careful to make a thorough study of the water availability and needs in both the Owens Valley and Los Angeles. His studies on California water were published in the Geological Survey's Annual Reports for 1898, and he discussed it thoroughly with his superior in Washington. He argued that the water should be used where it would do "the greatest good for the greatest number." The idea was passed up the line to President **Theodore "Teddy" Roosevelt (1858-1909)** who endorsed the proposal with a public statement of its virtue. To be sure, "the greatest good for the greatest number" has the moral equivalent of something like Robin Hood's "steal from the rich and give to the poor," but it seemed to make sense and had political appeal.

William Mulholland was placed in charge of building the aqueduct. Born in 1855 in Belfast, Ireland, he had gone to sea in his youth and had crossed the ocean 19 times before jumping ship in America. His first experience with fresh water was hand drilling artesian wells in Compton, and later as a ditch tender at $1.50 a day for the Los Angeles Water Company that supplied the city with water from the Los Angeles River. Mulholland rose rapidly in the company to become superintendent in 1886 at $500 a month. In his spare time he read extensively on a wide range of subjects, and truly a self-educated man, he gained membership in the American Society of Engineers in 1907.

Mulholland calculated that the aqueduct would cost $23 million, and the city voted bonds to raise $25 million. The aqueduct was a major undertaking that sluiced Owens River water into a canal, tunnel, and a huge steel pipe to siphon the water over the hills. Mulholland demonstrated exceptional engineering and management skills, bringing the complicated project to conclusion at a cost of about $24.5 million. On November 5,

1913, the gates were opened and a cascade of melted Sierra snow gushed down a trough into a canal that flowed to the San Fernando Reservoir, providing moisture for thousands of new homes, lawns, swimming pools, golf courses, tree-lined streets and parks, and cooling for power plants that energized blazing lights and air conditioners. Water for irrigation blanketed the San Fernando Valley with orchards of oranges and lemons. The melted mountain snow created dozens of millionaire Realtors, developers and financial institutions, leaving the once-luscious Owens Valley desolate and bare, with enraged residents having little recourse but to litigate in the legal bramble of riparian rights. Mulholland was widely acclaimed for the accomplishment, having his name among many other honors on a school, a drive, and a monument.

The city's Faustian bargain paid off in spades, but the Devil had an ace up his sleeve. The irresistible attraction of warm winters and sunny skies to easterners and mid-westerners fed up with cold and clammy winters induced an influx of people faster than public facilities could be provided, resulting in congestion, air pollution—the worst in the nation—from the exhaust of automobiles and trucks containing poisonous ozone, carcinogenic benzene, and carbon monoxide. Unhealthful particulate smog gave visual evidence of its spread throughout much of the Los Angeles basin westward as far as the ocean and eastward through the Banning pass, bleeding into the desert to Palm Springs and beyond. The molasses-like traffic on major arteries spawned the mental disorder "road rage," sometimes culminating in violence. The health effects of such stressful living remain to be fully documented.

But Los Angeles was not through quenching its thirst. In 1940 it invested $40 million to extend the aqueduct 40 miles farther north to tap into the streams flowing into Mono Lake. In 1970 it invested $88 million to construct a second aqueduct that doubled the ability to deliver water from the Mono Basin and Owens Valley. The Los Angeles Department of Water and Power (LADWP) is now the largest municipal utility in the country, getting some of the water from as far north as the Sacramento-San Joaquin delta of San Francisco Bay and as far east as the Colorado River. The LADWP provides services to 680,000 water customers and 1.4 million electric customers.

On July 11, 2007, after nearly 100 years of contentious litigation involving a variety of interests, Superior Court Judge **Lee F. Cooper** approved an agreement between LADWP, Inyo County, Department of Fish and Game, State Lands Commission, Owens Valley Committee, and the Sierra Club in which LADWP agreed to establish flow on the Owens River in perpetuity. Water started to flow again permanently for 62 miles along the Owens River bed to where it is diverted back into the aqueduct for use of the LADWP.

Health would be better in the Los Angeles Basin today if the city had been as visionary in supporting "The World's Greatest Electric Railway System" as in providing water. The Pacific Electric Railway (PE) was built during 1900 to 1910 by **Henry Edwards Huntington** (1850-1927) whose uncle, **Collis Potter Huntington** (1821-1900) helped finance the Central Pacific Railroad, which linked with the Union Pacific in 1869 to become the first transcontinental railroad.[2] Henry's PE at its peak in the 1920s advertised "1000 miles of Standard Trolley Lines" and 2,700 scheduled trains daily. PE operated 900 cars, called "big red cars" on routes that extended over Los Angeles, Orange, San Bernardino, and Riverside Counties, skirting the beaches, into the mountains, linking hundreds of towns and farmlands.[3, 4] But, the popularity of the automobile had come into play in a big way around 1912. Roads and highways were cheap and easy to build across land covered with sage brush, or blanketed with open fields of beans and sugar beets. Privately owned and maintained railways could not keep fares low enough to compete with free government-built roads. Federal subsidies of railways had been handed out in support of transcontinental railroads when they were given huge blocks of land—alternate square miles (640 acres)—along the right of way. But there was no help or even sympathy for the PE. Big players in the automobile, gasoline, and tire industries were accused of slick lobbying for cars and buses. Maybe they did, but the truth is that trolleys could not compete with the glamor of speeding on the open highway. PE revenue reached a peak in 1923 and declined to an operating loss in 1931, surging briefly in days of World War II to a record profit in 1943, followed by annual losses until the end came in 1953 when only a few cars remained. Los Angeles and outlying cities and residential areas are now in desperate need of reliable, rapid transportation as a way to reduce congestion and emissions of smog and greenhouse gases. The PE, which could have been a partial solution and a strong beginning for something even better, is a vanished dream.

Water for Los Angeles' neighbor, arid Orange County, was just as critical and more complicated. During agricultural development of the area, shallow wells, some of them artesian, provided an abundance of irrigation water for the expansive fields of beans, beets, and other crops. Unfortunately, the underground water was from an aquifer that extended under the ocean. Withdrawal brought an intrusion of salt water into the water supply even after residential development led to all the wells being capped except those used for the domestic supply. Since 1975 the county has been purifying sewer water and injecting it into the aquifer as a partial barrier to salt water intrusion. The water district with the help of several agencies is spending $450 million on a groundwater replenishment (GWR) system, which they boast of as being the largest water purification system of its kind in the world. It will take highly treated sewer water and further purify it to meet state and federal drinking water standards—as pure as bottled water. Purification is done in a stepwise process that includes reverse osmosis (also used by some suppliers of bottled water), micro filtration with ultraviolet light, and hydrogen peroxide oxidation. The process is cheaper than sea water desalination. The water is then injected into the groundwater basin or into deep aquifers as an underground barrier to ocean water intrusion. There it will become part of the drinking water supply. About half of the purified water will be piped to upstream lakes where it will follow the path of rainwater by filtering through the clay, sand, and rock to deep aquifers of the groundwater basin. The main source for that purpose is water from the Santa Ana and Colorado Rivers.

CHAPTER 26

FEEDERS AND BREEDERS

When our remote ancestors engaged in the adventure of becoming human a million or so years ago they managed to feed themselves barely enough to keep their numbers ahead of a stable population, probably increasing no more than .001 percent a year. When they invented agriculture about 10,000 years ago, their numbers increased dramatically, leading to civilization and the convenience of specialties. Farming evolved from subsistence agriculture to become the most basic specialty in a society of feeders and breeders. The abundance and variety of food led to better health and longer life. The human population is now increasing at the rate of about 1.7 percent a year. It was estimated to have reached 7 billion in 2011.

The breeders are winning the game in numbers but losing in the quality of life. Catastrophe was predicted in 1798 by **Thomas Robert Malthus** (1766-1834), an Englishman who as a young man entered the ministry but switched careers, becoming the first professor of economics when he took a position to train young executives of the East India Company. Shortly after graduating from Cambridge University, he published anonymously a treatise entitled *Essay on Population* in which he said that people of the world would outbreed their capacity to feed themselves. Malthus was scorned by many people as a pessimistic visionary, but it turned out that his prediction was close to the truth. To be sure, most of us who live in advanced parts of the world where soil and water are abundant and the earth is tilled by modern methods are well fed. But vast areas of the world with marginal soil and water are overpopulated and underfed. **David Pimintel and Marcel Pimintel**, food and agriculture scholars at Cornell University, give an estimate that 1 to 2 billion people are malnourished, roughly up to a third of the 7 billion people on earth.[1] According to Norman Borlaug, 800 million people experience chronic and transitory hunger,[2] and 25,000 people are said to die every day of malnutrition.

Lester R. Brown could be seen as a reincarnation of Malthus, except Brown saw the balance between population and food in relation to the impact of people on the environment. Brown is the former President and Founder of the Worldwatch Institute in which for 3 years he helped pioneer the idea of environmental sustainable development for food production. In 2001 he founded the Earth Policy Institute "to provide a vision of an environmental sustainable economy—an eco-economy—along with a roadmap of how to get from here to there." He has authored or coauthored some 50 books, printed in some 40 languages, and has received several awards including the Presidential Medal of Italy, and honorary professor at the University of Shanghai.

In his book, *Outgrowing the Earth*, Lester Brown emphasizes the critical problems of water supply for crop irrigation and stabilizing the declining underground water table. Water supplies are perilous not only in desert areas but also in high use areas where the aquifers are being rapidly depleted. Falling water tables together with rising global temperatures will require more efficient ways to water crops. Drip irrigation and other methods to ration the delivery of water will have to be increasingly implemented.[3] The National Geographic dramatized the problem by devoting a special issue to *Water: Our Thirsty World*, April 2010.

Agriculture now uses 70 percent of the available fresh water that is increasingly used by the proliferation of suburbs in and around expanding cities. There is an ever-growing demand for domestic water for household use, swimming pools, lawns, golf courses, parks, and landscaping. The arid southwest of the United States is in conflict. We have seen what happened when the city of Los Angeles surreptitiously acquired nearly all the water rights in the Owens Valley, piped the Owens River snow-melt from the High Sierras to the faraway mega-city, leaving the once-lush farmland a barren dusty desert. In recent years, Las Vegas, Nevada and the surrounding area have had the most rapid housing buildup in the nation, drawing most of their water from the Colorado River, desperately needed elsewhere for agricultural use. Expansion of housing continues in the Coachella Valley of California. An aerial view of the valley, including Palm Springs, is a giant blue and green checkerboard of swimming pools, lawns, and golf courses. Water comes by canal from the Colorado River. It's called the All American Canal because it crosses over the Mexico border and back to avoid some hilly sand dunes. Domestic users can pay much more for water than farmers can afford. An alarming example is the contract negotiated with the Imperial Valley Water District to buy from agreeing farmers their rights to Colorado River water, which would be transported over ranges of mountains to the city of San Diego. The result: some of the most productive vegetable-growing land in the country will be returned to the desert.

The food supply has increased over time but it has been a struggle to keep pace with population growth. World grain production was 1.1 tons per hectare in 1950 and increased to 2.9 tons per hectare by 2004. Expectation of a large increase in population led to efforts to further increase productivity by stepped up crop subsidies, research, extension services, and more use of fertilizers, insecticides and weed killers.

Norman E. Borlaug (1914-2009) was a pioneer in developing ways to increase and stabilize the world's food supply. While with the Rockefeller Foundation's agriculture team in Mexico he spearheaded a plant breeding research project on varieties of stem rust resistant wheat, said to be the world's largest planted acreage of food crops. Within 12 years of improving seeds and agronomic practices Borlaug's team increased Mexican wheat production five-fold, according to **Christopher Dowswell**'s *retrospective*.[4] Borlaug's Green Revolution added hundreds of millions of tons of grain to world harvests and is credited with saving hundreds of millions of lives. He was awarded the Nobel Peace Prize in 1970. The citation read, "More than any other single person of this age, he has helped to provide bread for a hungry world."

Borlaug grew up on a farm near Cresco, Iowa, with thoughts of becoming a high school science teacher but ended up devoting his professional life to providing food for hungry people of the world. He enrolled at the University of Minnesota in 1932. It was at the height of the Great Depression, and Borlaug could never forget the sight of people camped in parks, desperately hungry and begging for food. In 1937, he heard a lecture by **Elvin Stakman**, a prominent plant pathologist at the University who had worked on ways to deal with stem rust of wheat, epidemics of which periodically devastated wheat fields around the world. Borlaug was so inspired that he switched to plant pathology and obtained his doctoral under Stakman in 1942. He served during the war as a microbiologist working on fungicides and bactericides for the Du Pont Company, and in 1944 went to Mexico to join Stakman who was working on the Rockefeller Foundation's program to improve wheat production. During Borlaug's work there he trained a team of scientists in plant breeding, selection of seeds, and agronomic methods. He made a practice of educating both students and farmers in the use of fertilizers, pest control and irrigation. He was called upon for help in Asia and Africa under the auspice of the newly created International Maize and Wheat Improvement Center. Borlaug's team made thousands of crosses of wheat varieties from around the world to determine if they were adaptable to differences in soil, climate and other local conditions.[5]

In 1985 a Japanese philanthropist **Ryoichi Sasakawa** proposed an agricultural extension program for some of the African countries. A Sasakawa-Global 2000 agricultural program began operating in 15 sub-Saharan countries. Borlaug was greeted with the same enthusiasm as in Mexico and Asia, but he found conditions in Africa more difficult. Lack of roads, railroads, electricity, irrigation systems, fertilizer, and supply outlets made it unlikely that an African Green Revolution would materialize soon. Another problem arose that could threaten the worldwide supply of wheat. The fungus that causes stem rust of wheat had been beaten down in Mexico by Borlaug's expertise in plant breeding that established rust-resistant strains of the grain. But a new virulent and aggressive variety of rust fungus that causes what is called yellow rust (also known as stripe rust) spread rapidly and reached epidemic proportions in several countries on five continents since 2000. The yellow rust epidemic hit the United States and Australia, and devastated wheat growing areas of China, northern and eastern Africa, eastern and central Asia, and the Middle East. Yellow rust has some virulent strains that are high-temperature tolerant and are believed to be still evolving.[6] As Norman Borlaug said, "Rust never sleeps."

An action of the United States to reduce vehicle air pollution dealt a blow to scientists and agriculturalists who had labored for years to feed a hungry world. In the 1990s Congress amended the Clean Air Act with legislation that said gasoline used in specified heavily air-polluted areas must contain at least 2% oxygen. The purpose of oxygen is to promote complete combustion of polluting hydrocarbons instead of releasing the unburnt poisons, along with ozone, into the air. An oxygenate called MTBE (methyl tert-butyl ether), suspected of being a carcinogen, had been used for the purpose for many years, but was banned by several states due to contamination of ground water from leaking tanks.[7] The oil companies had to do something quickly. They seized on ethanol (ordinary ethyl alcohol like that in beer, wine and whiskey) for which there was an abundant supply of raw material—**corn**. It was a turning point in what **Donald Kennedy**, former Editor-in-chief of *Science*, called the "biofuels craze."[8] Other critics referred to it as "fuel from food."

The 2% oxygen requirement could be met by blending gasoline with about 5 to 10 percent ethanol. Most of the ethanol is sold for use as an additive to gasoline. But in the Midwest, much of it is sold as E85 (85% ethanol, 15% gasoline) requiring engine modifications. Replacement of gasoline with ethanol, advocates said, would reduce pollution and greenhouse gases from auto exhausts, and besides, would ease the country's reliance on imported oil and encourage the use of biofuels. Politicians saw still another advantage. A subsidy for ethanol from corn would further cement relations with a segment of society favored by Washington since before the dust bowl days depicted in *Grapes of Wrath*. Congress enacted legislation that provided a federal excise tax exemption of 5.1 cents per gallon for fuel blended with 10% ethanol, making the subsidy 51 cents per gallon of ethanol. To block competition from cheaper Brazilian ethanol made from sugar cane Congress imposed a tariff of 54 cents a gallon of ethanol. Brazil is a logical source of ethanol not only because it has a vast subtropical area with a climate and water supply ideal for growing sugar cane but also, during fermentation yeast produces alcohol from cane sugar without the need for adding an expensive enzyme to convert starch to a sugar as required for fermenting ethanol from corn. Besides, cane will produce more than twice as much ethanol per acre as corn. Early in the game, Brazil's dictator, General **Ernesto Geisel**, subsidized and financed ethanol plants and ordered the state-owned oil company to install tanks and pumps to supply users. Today nearly all cars sold in Brazil run exclusively on ethanol.[9] Unfortunately, the demand for new land in Brazil promotes cutting and clearing forests at a rate that creates several environmental problems including an increase in greenhouse gases that threaten global climate.

California answered the siren call to cash in on making ethanol. The state is not noted for growing yellow feed corn, but it could, because it has large beef feed lots. The largest of four companies that entered the fray, eligible for up to $15 million in subsidies, was Pacific Ethanol founded by former California secretary of state, **Bill Jones**, a Republican party stalwart who had given $70,000 to governor **Arnold Schwarzenegger**'s campaign. Pacific Ethanol filed for bankruptcy protection in 2009 but the California Energy Commission promised to bail out the struggling company with millions of dollars to be made available with a fund provided by the legislature entitled Alternate Fuel and Vehicle Technology Program. The author of the bill, former Assembly Speaker **Fabian Nunez** cried foul. "It's appalling," he was quoted by *Los Angeles Times* reporter **Jack Dolan**. "We gave then a very clear direction where these funds should be going. Ethanol is yesterday's news. It seems like there's some inside deal going on."[10]

Some highly qualified scientists who made calculations on the value of using ethanol as a gasoline additive showed that there was a net negative energy balance. In short, making ethanol from corn uses more energy, much of it from petroleum, than it produces. **Tad W. Patzek**, professor of civil and environmental engineering at the University of California, Berkeley, who devoted two years to a study of the energy input of ethanol, was quoted, "In terms of renewable fuels, ethanol is the worst solution. It has the highest energy cost with the least benefit." He declared that using ethanol as a gasoline additive results in a net energy loss of 65%. He pointed out that those who claim an energy gain from ethanol do not account for the energy it takes to produce corn and ethanol—cultivation of soil, water, disposal of waste water, pesticides, herbicides, hauling, use of tractors and trucks, building and operating fermentation and distillation plants. Besides, ethanol is so corrosive that it cannot be transported over gasoline pipelines, so it must be carried by trucks or rail, all adding to the cost. **David Pimintel**, professor emeritus of ecology at Cornell University is just as adamant about the ethanol-gasoline energy balance. He said, "Biofuels are total waste and misleading us from getting at what we really need to do: conservation…. Many people are seeing this as a boondoggle." Most of the people who have a financial interest in ethanol, also the U.S. department of Agriculture, claim that there is an energy gain in making ethanol from corn. Pimentel, a relentless critic, was quick to point out that their calculations failed to factor in some of the production costs.[11]

The U.S. Department of Agriculture surveyed 86,000 farmers and calculated that they would plant 90.5 million acres of corn in 2007. More would follow. A 2007 energy bill mandated an increase in biofuels five-fold to 36 billion gallons by 2022. Farmers reduced soybean acreage to make land available for corn. Nearly all the ethanol made in the U.S. is made from yellow feed corn. The distilleries compete with meat producers for feed corn, driving up the price. The stampede to convert land from other crops to plant more corn, build ethanol plants, step up fertilizer production, and require more seed such as Monsanto's gene-engineered herbicide-resistant seed was reminiscent of the California gold rush of 1849, but more profitable to more people.[12] It was a disaster for millions of people living on subsistence diets in other parts of the world. The price of corn that had been stable at around $2 a bushel jumped to $6 a bushel. Wheat went up 86 percent. Soy beans went up 93 percent. The World Bank estimated that food prices soared 83% in three years.[13] In Mexico, the birthplace of the Green Revolution, corn is a staple. So are tortillas. They don't taste as good without cornmeal, but with it now they cost more.

Days of prosperity and promise for ethanol producers began to fade within five years of the giddy days when government subsidies and mandates stimulated a lucrative increase in corn crops and construction of plants to process the production of ethanol. An extended drought had reduced the corn crop to the point where commodity prices were pushed so high that ethanol was too expensive to produce. By 2012 nearly 10% of the country's ethanol plants had stopped production. The communities that prospered from growing corn and engaged in the production, storage, and dealing with ethanol suffered.

Thousands of barrels of ethanol remained in storage because there was not enough gasoline being used to blend it with. Related activities suffered. Farmers have to deal with local merchants in various ways. They buy feed and equipment for livestock. Travelers and truck drivers give some relief by dealing with restaurants, hotels and banks. The future for ethanol remains to be seen. One unknown is the popularity of smaller automobiles and those that use less fuel. Natural gas is another option that remains to be exploited as a replacement for gasoline.

According to a National Research Council report, the United States could reduce the use of fossil fuel by 80% by 2050 in light duty cars and trucks. This could be done, the report said, by the use of more efficient vehicles, reduction in the use of gasoline combined with alternative fuels such as electricity, biofuels, and hydrogen. Such developments would drastically reduce the need for ethanol.[14, 15]

The US federal and state governments were key players in feeding the people of the young country when it was essentially an agricultural economy even before the establishment of land-grant colleges and universities by the Land Grant Act of 1862 under which Congress granted in each case 30,000 acres of land to be sold and the proceeds used to create and maintain a college or university to teach the fine points of agriculture and the mechanical arts. The states and territories received a total of 11,367,832 acres of land for the purpose. Today, every state and Puerto Rico receive federal grants to support land-grant colleges and universities, many of which over time became prestigious research universities such as Illinois, Texas, Washington, and California.

And that is not all. Various crop subsidies, grants, farm loans, crop rotation and development of varieties were among measures to help farmers. A classic example is the so-called Sugar Subsidy Battle. Legislation enacted by Congress required that at least 85% of sugar sold in the United States must come from domestic processors. Sugar supplies are managed by the U.S. Department of Agriculture that informs sugar producers how much sugar they can sell and limits how much can be imported. They can also buy up excess sugar and sell it to ethanol makers, even at a loss. In May, 2012, raw sugar sold for 30.2 cents a pound on the U.S. market and 20.5 cents a pound on the world market. Refined sugar sold for 59.5 cents a pound on the U.S. market and 25.5 cents a pound on the world market. Much of the sugar business is on the west coast with a sugar cane processing plant, American Sugar Refining, in Crockett in the San Francisco Bay area of California and a sugar beet refinery in Brawley, California.

Candy and gum makers, bakers, and other sugar users are bracing for a bitter fight, contending that the government should get out of the sugar business. The battle is over a farm bill that would renew the sugar program.[16]

The severe drought in the United States during the 2012 season caused the corn crop to wither and livestock to suffer from scarcity and high cost of food. The U.S. Department of Agriculture announced that it would buy up to $170 million worth of meat from affected livestock producers. They said that the purchase of $100 million in pork, $10 million in lamb, $50 million in chicken, and $10 million in catfish would provide some relief. The USDA had previously allowed the farmers to obtain expedited low interest emergency loans.[17, 18]

All this suggests that U.S. lawmakers are determined to give agricultural segments of the economy extraordinary help, a carryover from an earlier time when most Americans were making a hardscrabble living tilling the soil. Just as U.S. research universities are ranked by any standard among the best in the world and as such are incubators of the nation's prosperity, the variety, quality, and abundance of U.S. crop production, largely the result of Land-Grant Colleges and Universities, and the continued support of the U.S. government, is a marvel of the world. America's abundance has contributed to the nourishment in many parts of the world despite the monumental blunder of subsidizing the conversion of food to fuel that withdrew nearly 40 percent of the U.S. corn crop from the food and feed market to produce alcohol that could have been bought cheaper from Brazil as cane alcohol if not for a prohibitive U.S. tariff. At present, food donated to starving refugees in Africa comes mostly from the United States.

According to food and agriculture scholars, vast areas of the world are overpopulated and underfed. Cornell University's David and Marcel Pimintel said that roughly a third of the seven billion people on earth are malnourished. Lester Brown, founder of the Earth Policy Institute, spoke of critical problems related to a shortage of water supplies for crop irrigation in desert areas and in high use areas where aquifers are being depleted. Nobel Laureate Norman Borlaug, hero of the Green Revolution, said that 800 million people suffer from chronic hunger.

There are others who shrug off the pessimistic view that we are floundering in everlasting starvation and hunger. Instead, they say, people can breed and feed themselves far into the future. **H. Charles J. Godfrey**, zoologist at the University of Oxford, UK, thinks the number of people on earth is apt to top out at between 9 and 10 billion late in this century.[19]

A symposium on Feeding the World, organized by the Chemical Heritage Foundation, convened in November of 2011. Experts who attended the symposium predicted a sustainable food supply in a world that would probably contain 9 billion people by 2050.[20] **J. Vroom**, president and CEO of CropLife America, acknowledged some problems: weather and climate change, government trade impediments, and economic instability. **Paul Rea** of BASF Crop Protection USA, pointed out that 40% of crops are lost to pests, weeds, and diseases in the face of millions of dollars invested and years in development that are needed to bring a product to market. **Antonio Galindez** president and CEO of Dow Agroscience said that his company invests $6 billion annually in creating agricultural products that probably will not show results until 2025.

Keynote speaker **Matt Ridley**, author of *The Rational Optimist*, contended that irrigation, crop protection products, and other techniques have reduced the amount of land needed to produce crops.[21] He could have mentioned that adding two or three billion people to the population would reduce food production by urbanizing thousands of acres of agricultural land. He could have mentioned that cutting tropical forests as in Brazil, and destroying the logs by burning, could adversely affect global climate. Much of the cleared land is used for cattle. Some, perhaps most, will be used for sugar cane to produce alcohol to replace all use of petroleum as fuel, reminiscent of the move by the United States where thousands of acres of corn were diverted from food to fuel, increasing the price of food in many parts of the world.

Ridley listed, without explaining, the scientific development that could have a major impact on world food production from *genetically modified seeds and plants*.

Monsanto Company embarked on the goal of developing corn seeds that would grow corn resistant to their blockbuster weed killer, *Roundup*, that is lethal to most species of broadleaf plants. The "Monsanto Magic" of genetically modified seeds was outstandingly successful and highly profitable to Monsanto and corn farmers.[22] Other companies managed to intrude with a smaller stake in the method that Monsanto pioneered. The possibility that genetically modified crops might be successful in areas of extreme drought, extreme cold, extreme heat such as deserts, extremely short growing seasons, or ability to thrive in different soil types and fertility, could greatly expand the food supply of the world.[23]

Monsanto is not new to innovation. **John Queeny**, the founder of Monsanto Chemical Works in St. Louis, Missouri in 1901 used a horse or mule-drawn wagon for delivery from the factory of the artificial sweetener saccharin,[24] the sweetness of which was discovered by **Constantine Fahlberg**, a supervised student of an American chemist, **Ira Remsen**, (1846-1927) who patented the product.[25] Monsanto was probably the first American company to develop and commercialize aspirin. **Adolph Kolbe** (1818-1884), a German chemist who was an early synthesizer of organic compounds, made acetic acid from scratch and later made salicylic acid from salicin that led to the production of acetylsalicylic acid (aspirin)[26] which, therefore, can be said to be derived from the millennia-old medicine, salicin, abundant in the bark of white willow, *Salix alba* and related willows.[27]

PART VI
HUMANITY

27 Madness

28 Improving Mankind

29 Weeding The Unfit

30 The Master Race

31 Good From Evil

32 The Bargain

CHAPTER 27

MADNESS

Few things are more insane in the realm of health care than the historical treatment of the mentally ill. Nothing is more revealing of the paucity of human understanding and compassion than our treatment of those whose behavior deviates from the slippery standard of normal.

It's tempting to blame a shameful feature of human nature on something inherited from our ancestors. Even before they found comfort in caves, people crazy enough to deviate from the strict rules of conduct needed for survival of the family or tribe, no doubt would soon disappear, probably violently and devoid of sympathy. We see it in animals, for example, wild dogs and cats. In humans we see it repeated in history. Great thinkers who stir things up by advocating ways to overcome our more base animal inclinations are apt to pay the price of punishment, often death. Among hundreds of heroic victims were **Martin Luther King, Jr.** (1929-1968), **Mahatmas Gandhi** (1869-1948), and **Jesus of Nazareth**, the latter executed by the method of cruelty prevailing at the time. None of these men were mentally impaired. Thousands of heretics were burned at the stake during the Inquisition. **Galileo** (1564-1642) escaped with his life, though spending his last years under house arrest. **Giordano Bruno** (1548-1600), an Italian scholar noted for his work in physics and astronomy, was burned alive at the stake. He had traveled a lot and talked a lot, agreeing with the calculations of **Nicolas Copernicus** (1473-1543) about the solar system and believed, as did **Nicolas of Cusa** (1401-1464) an astronomer of a century and a half earlier, that the sun is at the center of the solar system, that the universe is infinite, and that the stars are suns that support other inhabitable planets. Bruno was imprisoned in Rome for seven years, tried and convicted of heresy, apostasy, blasphemy, and misconduct and put to his death in flames on February 17, 1600. Holding to his intellectual integrity to the end, he refused to accept the cross held out to him at the last moment.

People living in large groups had to find a way to isolate mentally deviant members by caring for them at home or, if violent or obstreperous, keeping them locked in a room or building. In the early Middle Ages hospitals were for the physically sick, not for people believed to be possessed of devils. The latter were locked up in chains, naked in unheated buildings, poorly fed, beaten when their anguished cries annoyed their keepers, and left in their excrement until they died. In England the hospital of St. Mary of Bethlehem was founded in 1247 and by the fifteenth century came to be specialized as a lunatic asylum. Noted for its barbaric treatment of the inmates, it became notorious as Bethlem, better known as "Bedlam." Charles Dickens referred to it in *David Copperfield*, "It's a mad world. Mad as Bedlam." Bedlam became a showplace of London where visitors came to be entertained by viewing the inmates. At other asylums in Europe, as well, where the inmates were kept in cages, visitors were charged an entrance fee.

Display of the mentally ill for amusement continued well into the nineteenth century. The victims were still commonly held in chains but over time treatment became less brutal. Inmates were sometimes treated with drugs such as opium to calm them, while the standard "curative" was frequent bleeding. A pioneer in attempts to improve the treatment of inmates was **Philippe Pinel** (1745-1826), a physician at the Hopital Bicere in France. It was shortly after the French Revolution (1789-1799), whose leaders found lavish use of the invention of **Joseph Guillotin** (1738-1814). (Antoine Lavoisier, a brilliant French chemist called the father of modern chemistry, was guillotined on May 8, 1794, by the revolutionary leaders. It is said that when Lavoisier protested that he was only a scientist, the arresting officer replied, "The Republic has no need for scientists." Probably the reason Lavoisier was guillotined was because he had made the mistake of investing in a firm, of which his father-in-law was an executive, that was engaged in tax collecting. The tax collectors were permitted to keep anything they could collect above the actual tax. The lucrative business was called "tax farming," resented with a passionate hatred. Lavoisier's father-in-law and other tax farmers were also guillotined.)[1] It was still risky to upset the apple cart with bold moves, so Pinel requested permission of authorities to treat the inmates more humanely. He removed the chains, fed them better, and improved the deplorably unsanitary conditions.

In the United States most of the mentally ill were held in poor houses or jails. **Dorothea Lynde Dix** (1802-1887) was superintendent of Women Nurses for the Union during the Civil War, and was instrumental in establishing numerous state asylums which greatly improved the conditions of the mentally ill. She also led a drive to improve the treatment in prisons. Dix was born in Hampden, Maine, but grew up in Massachusetts. When she visited a house of correction in 1841 she was shocked by the treatment of the mentally ill people. She implored legislators in Massachusetts to provide better care for them and started her reform movement in that state. She traveled widely in the U.S. and Europe, and was able to get the support of wealthy people, distinguished educators, and statesmen, continuing to promote the cause until she was 80 years old.

Many of the asylums were built on expansive grounds believed to have a beneficial effect, but they could be gloomy places to live in. The Danvers State Hospital in Massachusetts, was built in 1841 and closed in 1955. Journalist **Nellie Bly** spent time undercover in the hospital in 1887 and wrote that it was a "human rat trap." There was a movement to close asylums and to place the inmates in smaller homes or hospitals. After the Danvers Hospital was closed, the abandoned building, described as "the scariest building in the world" became a favorite of thrill-seeking ghost hunters.

The twentieth century experienced the most extreme treatment of mental illness since prehistoric times. In prehistory we see in museums human skulls, of people who lived thousands of years ago, with rectangular holes in them showing precise cuts. Some damage to the brain was inevitable but there is no way of knowing whether parts of the brain were deliberately removed. It was the earliest known surgical operation, now called *Trephining* for making a hole in a bone with a modern instrument called a trephine or trepan. Trephining was practiced by tribes of the American Indians, and until recently, tribes of North Africa and Melanesia are known to have practiced it as healing magic. Maybe some still do. What better way would there be to allow the demons of the brain to escape?

The first in a modern setting to revive the millennia-old savagery of cutting into the skull was in 1888 when **Gottlieb Burckhardt**, a Swiss asylum superintendent, removed brain tissue from six patients. He reported the results at the Berlin Medical Conference. One of the patients died, others contracted leprosy, paralysis, or loss of ability to use or understand words. Interest in the procedure lagged until in 1935 **Antonio Egas Moniz**, professor of neurology in Lisbon, Portugal, witnessed the results of an experiment on two chimpanzees in which the frontal lobes had been removed, leaving them docile and vacant. He conducted similar operations to remove brain tissue from his human patients. He drilled holes in the patient's skulls and made cuts in the frontal lobes with a tool he called a "leucotome." It was reported that he declared the procedure "a stunning success" but a follow-up study revealed that his patients had relapses, seizures, and some deaths.[4]

The idea that the way to treat mental patients was to destroy part of the brain was enthusiastically promoted by an American psychiatrist, **Walter Freeman** (1895-1972). Freeman was not a licensed psychiatrist. After university schooling at Yale he entered Pennsylvania Medical School, then went to Europe to study neurology and psychiatry. On his return he set up private practice and joined the faculty at George Washington University as a professor of neurology where he was said to be a popular teacher. He engaged in radical experiments on mental patients such as giving massive doses of insulin and metrazol and administering high voltages of electroshock. He attended a presentation of the chimpanzee experiments and read of Moniz's experiments. He decided it was the answer. He ordered a supply of leucotomes and, together with a surgeon named **James Watt**, practiced on cadavers. They performed their first leucotomy on a 63 year-old Kansas woman who was suffering from insomnia and fits of hysteria. They drilled six holes into her head and cut the connections between the frontal lobes and the rest of the brain. Freeman proposed calling the operation "lobotomy." He was a showman, often calling reporters a day or two before a presentation at a medical conference. Watt complained that Freeman was like a barker at a carnival. Although many physicians were critical, the news stories were all laudatory. Freeman declared that "mental patients were better off without so much brain function". In a letter written by Freeman to a patient in a malpractice suit he warned her to go to a hospital because in checking on his post-lobotomy patients around the country he found that many of them had committed suicide. The patient in this case had suffered severe dementia involving loss of intellect and emotional functioning.

Freeman read about an Italian surgeon who entered the brain through the eye socket. He liked the idea of performing a lobotomy by a method that would avoid cutting a hole through the skull. Freeman decided that the least intrusive way was to use an ice pick and called the procedure "transorbital lobotomy." He started doing the operation in his office: no cutting, no drilling, no surgeon, no anesthesiologist, no hospital stay, almost no recovery time. He would put the patients on a table, knock them out with electroshock, insert the ice pick through the eye socket, and swing the pick back and forth making slices in the frontal lobes. He could complete the operation in 15 minutes, making no effort to use sterile methods. He perfected the technique with a flamboyant demonstration of holding an icepick in each hand and inserting them in both sockets at the same time. He visited state hospitals around the country, treating many patients per day. He said that during his career he conducted 5,000 lobotomies. He was awarded honors for his work by his colleagues and became director of neurology and psychiatry at George Washington University.

Peter Sterling, a neuroanatomist at the University of Pennsylvania in an article in New Republic of March 3, 1979, entitled *Psychiatry's Drug Addiction*, pointed out a similarity in effect of lobotomy to that of some powerful drugs.

A glimpse of the results of lobotomy was seen in the movie based on Ken Kesey's 1962 book, *One Flew Over the Cuckoo's Nest* in which Jack Nicholson, playing the part of the patient, McMurphy, is given an electric shock treatment, and when that fails to restrain a violent outburst of disgust and indignation brought on by a supervisor's cruel and abusive treatment of a patient, it is followed with a lobotomy. A patient-friend is so upset on seeing McMurphy brought back like a depersonalized zombie, that he puts McMurphy out of his misery by suffocating him with his pillow, then escapes into the night by crashing through a window.

Psychosurgery for treatment of obsessive-compulsive disorder came to be favored by some psychiatrists. **Michael Jenike**, director of the Obsessive-Compulsive Disorder Clinic and Research Unit at the Massachusetts General Hospital was quoted as speaking highly of a form of lobotomy, called "cingulotomy," in which electrodes inserted into the brain electrically melts the nerve connections to the frontal lobes. The main surgeon at the hospital, **H.T. Ballantine**, performed hundreds of cingulotomy operations, mostly on women, and for a variety of ailments, including back pain. He said that he believed the operation corrected biochemical imbalances.[5]

Some of the work in psychosurgery appears to have been racially motivated. Experiments were conducted at the University of Mississippi in Jackson on emotionally distressed and abandoned African American children. The director of neurosurgery, **O. J. Andy**, would insert multiple electrodes into the brains of children as young as five. Experiments would sometimes be repeated several times over periods of months or years to determine the outcome in older children or even as adults. At about the same time, Harvard Medical School's neurosurgeons **Vernon Mark** and **William Sweet** implanted dozens of electrodes in the brains of patients as an attempt to cure violence. They thought that black urban rioters had a brain disease that could be cured by brain surgery.[6]

It appears that by now most psychosurgery has been discontinued. Belief in the value of lobotomy waned while at the same time an interest developed in various forms of shock treatment.

In 1972, **Peter R. Breggin**, an American psychiatrist, organized an international campaign to stop the return of lobotomy and other forms of psychosurgery. He conducted a decades-long campaign against electroshock treatment. Breggin was trained at Harvard College and Case Western Reserved Medical School, took his residence at the Massachusetts Mental Health Center, and became a full-time consultant with the National Institute of Mental Health (NIMH). He left in 1968 to go into private practice as a psychiatrist. He became Director of the International Center for the Study of Psychiatry and Psychology, and founder and co-editor of *Ethical Human Sciences and Services.*

An early shock treatment was to drop the naked patient into a tank of cold water. That treatment was superceded by "insulin coma." Metropolitan State Hospital in Massachusetts had an insulin coma room where rows of patients were overdosed with insulin causing a rapid drop in blood sugar to the point where they fell into convulsions, then coma from starvation of the brain. A young medical student who later became a psychiatrist, wrote, "As I watched them writhe about on mats, near death, it seemed like a scene from hell. The once difficult and unruly inmates, with their brains now permanently damaged, became gratefully dependent on their keepers after being brought back from the edge of death.[7]

Another treatment was to infect the patient with malaria which, by inducing fever, was believed to improve the condition of patients with paresis, an advanced debilitating form of syphilis that impaired functions of the brain and nervous system.

With a decline in the use of the objectionable lobotomy there was a continuing interest in electroconvulsive therapy, better known as electroshock treatment. It was first tried in 1938 by an Italian psychiatrist, **Ugo Cerletti** (1877-1963) who was head of Mental and Neurological Diseases at the University of Rome. The procedure is to place electrodes on the frontoparietal regions of the head and apply a voltage discharge.

A newer way to alter brain function with electric currents is by a method called transcranial magnetic stimulation (TMS) in which a technician places a ring-shaped so-called paddle near the scalp, and when the electricity is turned on, currents swirling inside the paddle create a magnetic field which in turn generates currents in the brain tissue. Since transmission of signals along a nerve fiber are accomplished by a chemically induced electric impulse from neuron to neuron, the magnetic field disrupts that electrical activity. Although thousands of people have been given TMS in clinical trials to treat psychiatric problems, especially depression, it is not clear exactly how it works. Despite the gaps in knowledge of what it does to the brain, The Food and Drug Administration (FDA) took under consideration approval of TMS for daily use to treat depression.[9, 10]

By the late 20th century researchers had invented a variety of powerful antipsychotic drugs that calmed the patients and made them more docile. **Peter Sterling**, neuroanatomist at the University of Pennsylvania, wrote, "…lobotomies and chemicals like chlorpromazine may cause their effects in the same way, by disrupting the activity of the neurochemical, dopamine. At any rate, a psychiatrist would be hard-put to distinguish a lobotomized patient from one treated with chlorpromazine."[11] Chlorpromazine, one of the phenothiazine drugs, was the first drug to gain acceptance for treating a variety of psychosis related problems. It became one of the most widely used drugs in the practice of medicine.[12]

Authorities seized the opportunity to close some of the mental hospitals and send many of the inmates, along with newly diagnosed patients, home or to their communities as outpatients where they could be cared for and treated with the new drugs. It was a grand idea but there were unintended results. Many of the released patients have trouble adapting. Many refuse or evade taking the medicines, and become a burden on relief agencies, leaving thousands of our fellow beings to roam the streets homeless or hunker down under overpasses and alleys, many incompetent to be anything more than vagrants on skid row at the mercy of drug pushers, or locked up convicted of nonviolent victimless crimes such as possession of drugs or petty thievery to appease a drug addiction. Sentences are often out of proportion to the crime. A man suffering under a years-long bout of schizophrenia and convicted on charges related to scuffling with a security guard was sentenced to 35 years to life under the draconian three strikes law although one of the strikes was simply a threat with no physical contact. Thousands with undisclosed mental problems are thrown into overcrowded jails to mingle with vicious murderers, rapists, professional thieves, crooks, and gangsters where medical help for the mentally ill is not the top priority in a culture dominated by the political imperative of "tough on crime."

A study by the research arm of the U.S. Department of Justice concluded that large numbers of prison inmates suffer from depression, mania or other psychotic disorders. A survey of a sample of more than 25,000 prisoners nationwide found that mental health problems were related to the inmates record of violence and prior convictions. They were twice as apt to have been injured in prison fights, more likely to have been abused as children and homeless in the year before their arrest. Three-fourths of them were addicted to drugs or alcohol.

California keeps more people in jail than any other state. As of September, 2006, there were 172,000 inmates in the state's 33 prisons, 16,000 of them jammed into gymnasiums, hallways, or any space that could be found. Prison officials said that they would be out of room completely by the following summer. Such overcrowding makes recreational programs virtually impossible. It has been estimated that 20% to 25% of the inmates are bipolar, schizophrenic, clinically depressed, or otherwise mentally afflicted. The prison suicide rate in California is nearly twice the national average at 27 deaths per 100,000 inmates compared to the national average rate of 14 per 100,000. It's no surprise that California has the highest rate of recidivism in the country. A federal judge assigned to oversee the mental health problem in California's prisons ordered the immediate hiring of 550 psychiatrists and related mental health staff.[13]

Problems in California are not confined to state prisons. Juvenile facilities operated by the Probation Department of Los Angeles County erupted in race riots in 2005 and more than a dozen of the inmates escaped. Federal monitors found juvenile inmates shackled hand and foot for days on end. The monitors reported that juvenile inmates were not adequately screened for emotional or psychological problems.[14]

William McFarlane, a Psychiatrist at Maine Medical Center, is conducting a far-reaching study of *preventing* psychosis in those of greatest risk, called the Portland Identification and Early Referral (PIER) program. He works with communities in southern Maine on adolescents and young adults in crisis to prevent them from descending into profound mental illness. McFarlane believes that psychosis is preventable if caught early enough. Hallucinations, delusions, paranoia, schizophrenia, and other forms of psychotic illness afflict more than 2 million people in the United States and account for more than half the suicides among adolescents and young adults.[15]

The medical profession typically keeps a low profile on issues of public health. But it is in a position to bring change. In 2007, the American Medical Association (AMA) launched a three-year multimillion dollar campaign to promote its plan for health coverage for the estimated 45 million people in America who lack insurance. The AMA which represents about 250,000 physicians kicked off a "Voice for the Uninsured" ad campaign advocating tax credits or vouchers to help people buy health insurance as opposed to the idea of a government-run health insurance system. The initial drive directed $5 million in early primary states for radio, television, newspaper, and billboard advertising as well as pharmacy prescription bags and signs in mass transit conveyances. A second stage would expand the campaign to the entire country, and a third stage would lobby congressmen for legislation favoring the AMA's plan.

It may take a highly influential group of people similar to the AMA, with both the power to heal and the power to persuade, to break through the fog of apathy that is a drag on curing the combined mental health-juvenile-homeless-prisoner problems.

On March 23, 2010, Healthcare Reform was signed into law as the *Patient Protection and Affordable Care Act* also known as "Obamacare" after President Barack Obama. Designed to provide affordable health care for all US citizens, it requires the provision of many mandated services including preventative services as part of all health plans. The full implementation goes into effect in 2015 leaving the merits and shortcomings of this greatly debated legislation yet to be determined.

CHAPTER 28

IMPROVING MANKIND

The idea of improving certain characteristics of members of a tribe or nation has its roots in ancient Greece. The Spartans, physical fitness fanatics, encouraged wives of weaklings to mate with sturdy warriors. And **Julius Caesar** decreed that he had the right to mate with any married woman in the Empire. But it was not until the nineteenth century when a budding knowledge of heredity from animal breeding set the stage for European scientists to engage in a serious scrutiny of human heredity. In 1835 a Belgian astronomer and statistician, **Lambert Adolphe Jacques Quetelet** (1796-1874) recorded the chest measurements of Scottish soldiers and the height of French army draftees, as well as other physical characteristics. He plotted the results against the frequency of occurrence and found that they formed a bell-shaped curve. This form of statistical expression had been used so much by a famous German mathematician, **Johann Karl Friedrich Gauss** (1777-1855) that it is sometimes called a Gaussian curve, or more informally, a "normal" curve.

The desirability of manipulating human inheritance, and a way to accomplish it, attracted public attention by the work of an English anthropologist, Sir **Francis Galton** (1822-1911), a child prodigy who became a man of remarkably varied accomplishments. Born of a wealthy family and tutored by one of his sisters, he could read before he was three and was studying Latin at four. Among his many interests, he determined in 1869 that mental ability varied among people according to a bell shaped curve as had been shown by Quetelet to be true of physical characteristics. Galton was familiar with the pride taken by the landed gentry in raising pedigree livestock for prize-worthy characteristics. His cousin **Charles Darwin** (1809-1882) made a hobby of breeding pigeons. Galton had studied the intelligence of members of different families that gave evidence of the inheritance of intelligence, and this led him to take a strong position in the venerable argument over "nature versus nurture." He argued that desirable intellectual qualities of people could be increased by suitable breeding, and proposed the name *eugenics* to describe ways that it could be accomplished.[1]

We know now that breeding people for specific qualities would be more complex than Galton realized. He did not know about the studies on heredity of the Austrian botanist, **Gregor Mendel** (1822-1884) until late in his career, nor did he have the advantage of more recent knowledge of mutations, nor how a gene can vary in its effect on the development and performance of an organism according to discoveries in the newer science of *epigenetics*.

The idea of eugenic improvement was rejuvenated by an American geneticist, **Herman Joseph Muller** (1890-1967) who made important discoveries in mutations, especially ways to increase the mutation rate. Muller attended high school in the Bronx, New York, where he organized a science club. He entered Columbia University on a scholarship and continued graduate studies there under **Thomas Hunt Morgan** (1866-1945) who had introduced the technique of using *Drosophila*, the fruit fly, a tiny insect with only four pairs of chromosomes, for genetic studies. Fruit flies are easily cultured, have a short breeding cycle, and multiply in large numbers. Morgan's studies proved that chromosomes are the carriers of heredity and strongly supported an idea that genes determine individual characteristics. Morgan received the Nobel Prize in medicine and physiology in 1933.

Among several important discoveries, Morgan had observed many cases of mutations. Muller went a step further. He found that he could increase the mutation rate by irradiating the flies with X-rays. This led him to warn against the dangers of X-rays to humans. His knowledge of mutations and their causes and effects gave him concern about the welfare of people generally. He became active in publicizing the danger of increased mutations from the radioactive fallout from nuclear bomb tests. He was awarded the Nobel Prize in medicine and physiology in 1946.

Muller proposed eugenic measures to improve the genetic qualities of humans, and argued for the establishment of sperm banks to make the qualities of gifted men widely available. After Muller's death, a friend and admirer of Muller, wealthy businessman **Robert K. Graham**, established the Herman J. Muller Repository for Germinal Choice. Graham wrote to Nobel laureates asking for sperm donations, and five of them agreed. Many of them shrugged it off. **Linus Pauling** who won the 1954 Nobel Prize in chemistry and 1962 Nobel Prize for peace said that he preferred the old fashion way. But Graham received donations from other prominent scientists. The samples were kept as needed in a subterranean vault at his ten-acre estate near Escondido, California.

CHAPTER 29

WEEDING THE UNFIT

A forceful argument put forth by the defense in the Nuremberg trials was that the acts they were accused of were comparable to practices performed by and approved of over a period of years in the United States without penalty or prosecution. The presiding judge, United States Supreme Court justice **Robert H. Jackson** was undoubtedly aware of the history of the repulsive behavior of leaders of the medical, political and support community in the United States to which the German defense lawyers referred. But it did not diminish Justice Jackson's determination to bring the German criminals to justice.

The Germans on trial at Nuremberg could have made a more persuading defense if they could have known about the American abuses of prisoners during the Iraq war. Inhumane activities were not confined to experiments on patients. **Steven Miles**, a physician, describes in his book, *Oath Betrayed,* innumerable cases of torture of prisoners detained during the Iraq and Afghanistan wars, and the war against terror. Efforts to extract information, as well as torture seemingly only as entertainment were depicted in horrifying photos taken at the infamous Abu Ghraib army prison near Baghdad, seen worldwide. Dr. Miles asks, "Where were the doctors and nurses at Abu Ghraib?" He cited a passage in the Hippocratic Oath revered by doctors since 500 B.C.: "*I will use regimens for the benefit of the ill in accordance with my ability and my judgement but from what is to them harm or injustice I will keep them.*" People detained at the prison at Guantanamo Bay complained of torture. Many of the detainees were held for years without charges of guilt or without any effort to bring them to trial.

Almost nothing is known about the CIA and Special Forces interrogative centers in the war on terror in the Middle East, Asia, and

North Africa. The United States routinely refused to allow the Red Cross and UN monitors to interview prisoners privately about their treatment. And almost nothing is known about what happened to detainees who were secretly transported to Pakistan, Egypt, and Uzbekistan for imprisonment and interrogation. The CIA practice of sending detainees to other countries for imprisonment and interrogation was called "extraordinary rendition."[1]

Galton's emphasis on the distinction between nurture and nature, his legacy for establishment of the Eugenics Laboratory at the University of London, and the obvious conclusion that the quality of humanity could be improved by selective breeding as with livestock, fired the imagination of people on both sides of the Atlantic. The reduction of Galton's idea of eugenics to actual practice did not achieve much traction among the British because their main focus was on the positive aspect of selective breeding of superior individuals which they confidently thought was doing pretty well in their society. The practices in the United States referred to by the German defense lawyers was the result of the Americans' unrestrained enthusiasm for a distortion of Francis Galton's views. The American leaders in the eugenics movement were enthusiastic of what they perceived as a new and exciting science that was understandable to ordinary intelligent people. Their focus was on the negative aspect: preventing reproduction of the unfit who were contaminating the quality of humanity. The goal was pursued with unrestrained passion unequaled in science or society.

An influential proponent of improving the human race by sterilizing the unfit was **Dr. John H. Bell**, superintendent of Virginia Colony for Epileptics and Feeble-minded, who on October 19, 1927, performed the first operation under a 1926 act of the Virginia State Assembly that authorized sterilization of anyone determined to be mentally defective. The Virginia Colony had opened in 1910 under its first superintendent, **Dr. Albert S. Priddy**, who saw the institution as an opportunity to deal with the inherited causes of mental deficiency. In 1917 he asked the State Assembly to expand the purpose of the Colony to treat feeble-mindedness with surgical sterilization. A Virginia proposal in 1910 had been defeated although California had already legalized it. A 1916 revision of the law gave the superintendent governing Virginia Colony discretion to administer whatever medical and surgical treatment he deemed necessary. One of Dr. Priddy's treatments was to sterilize women for "pelvic disorders."

Dr. Bell was determined to get solid legal approval of sterilization by arranging for a challenge, hoping to take it to the Supreme Court. As a test case under the 1926 act of the state assembly he selected a 21-year old inmate, **Carrie Buck**. She had been assigned to the cafeteria where she might seem to most people to be a normal young woman. But Dr. Bell maintained that there was defect in her genes that made her promiscuous, a mother out of wedlock of a 3-year old daughter, clearly indicating that the woman was feebleminded. After being argued in state courts for three years, in 1927 the U.S. Supreme Court ruled 8 to 1 in *Buck vs. Bell* that the constitution did not prohibit compulsory sterilization. Writing the decision was assigned to Justice **Oliver Wendell Holmes, Jr.**, who expressed the predominant thinking of the time,

"*...It is better for all the world, if instead of waiting to execute degenerate offspring for crime, or to let them starve for their imbecility, society can prevent those who are manifestly unfit from continuing their kind. The principle that sustains compulsory vaccination is broad enough to cover cutting the Fallopian tubes....Three generations of imbeciles are enough.*" [2]

(On April 1, 2011, a gathering of legal scholars meeting at Pepperdine University's Law School announced that they had examined the U.S. Supreme Court's "Supreme Mistakes" and concluded that among the five worst decisions was the verdict in the 1927 trial of Buck vs. Bell which allowed sexual sterilization of institutionalized people without the patient's consent. The case was brought by Carrie Buck whom Dr. Bell had proclaimed feeble minded because she was promiscuous and had a child out of wedlock. He claimed that Carrie's mother and her three-year-old daughter were also mentally deficient. It was later divulged that the child resulted from Carrie Buck being raped by a family member of a caretaker.)[3]

Indiana was the first state to enact a law to authorize sterilization in 1907. California, the most aggressive in sterilization of all the states, enacted a similar law in 1909,[4] and by 1927, 15 more states enacted sterilization laws.

The most influential American disciple of Sir Francis Galton was **Charles Benedict Davenport**, who graduated from Harvard with a degree in theoretical science, taught at Harvard, then was appointed Assistant Professor at the University of Chicago. He was the first in the United States to teach the principles of heredity that had been discovered by Gregor Mendel. Eager to do research along those lines, in 1896 he persuaded the Carnegie Institution to fund what he called the Station for Experimental Evolution, at Cold Spring Harbor, a small town on the north shore of Long Island. Beginning in 1898 he conducted a popular Summer School at the Station. In 1906, through the influence of a student who was the daughter of Mrs. E. H. Harriman, wealthy widow of the railroad magnate **Edward Henry Harriman**, Davenport was able to persuade her to fund an expansion of the Station. Mrs. Harriman purchased an eighty acre property near the Station, was persuaded to pay for renovation of the Victorian house on it, and to fund the salaries of a superintendent and six workers, guaranteed for five years. The result, beginning in 1910, was the Eugenics Records Office to which Davenport appointed as director his energetic and enthusiastic protégée, **Harry Laughlin**, a Missouri school teacher. Davenport appointed a Board of Scientific Directors of the Records Office that included **Alexander Graham Bell**, the inventor, **Irving Fischer,** a professor at Yale, **William H. Welch** of Johns Hopkins, and **E.E. Southard** of Harvard.[5]

Research at the Station was focused on breeding experiments on a variety of animals from snails to chickens. Davenport's first project, seemingly inspired by Mendel's studies, was cross breeding chinch bugs, a small insect that thrives by sucking juice from grasses. It exists in two forms, long wing and short wing. In time, the Station at Cold Spring Harbor became one of the most prestigious research organizations in the country, attracting such luminaries as Nobel Laureate **James Watson**, co-discoverer of the structure of DNA, who for years served as director and leader in determining the human genome.

The initial impact, however, was from Laughlin's zeal, with Davenport's support, to stir up interest in eugenics, already a lively topic among the intelligentsia. He sent workers out to get thousands of pedigrees that could be used to evaluate the use of eugenics in relation to how the quality of Americans and humanity in general could be improved. His zeal got results. The House of Representatives committee on Immigration and Naturalization appointed Laughlin its Expert Eugenics Agent in which position he influenced the passage of a new law imposing new restrictions on immigration. He wrote a Model Sterilization Law under which the "unfit" could be sterilized without their consent. In his crusade to weed out the unfit and reproduce the fit he reached across the Atlantic, having an influence that later was to embarrass the United States prosecutors conducting the Nuremberg trials. **Adolf Hitler**'s Law for the Prevention of Genetically Diseased Offspring was patterned after Laughlin's model. Even before the Holocaust, over 150,000 Germans were forcibly sterilized. Heidelberg University gave Laughlin an honorary doctorate for his contributions to "racial hygiene."[6]

Meanwhile in the United States the corn flakes tycoon, **Dr. John Harvey Kellogg** of the Battle Creek Sanitarium amassed a fortune as an advocate of the healthy life. He decried the proliferation of lunatics, idiots, paupers, and other unfit people. There's an urgent need, he said, for genetic engineering. In apparent support for this thinking, President **Theodore Roosevelt** wrote in a letter to Davenport,"….we have no business to permit the perpetuation of citizens of the wrong type."[7]

CHAPTER 30

THE MASTER RACE

Adolph Hitler's (1889-1945) obsession with a supposed master race led him to his idea of eugenics as the way to maintain and improve the Aryan ideal. He urged strong, healthy young women, as a patriotic duty, to volunteer to mate with hand-picked officers of the Schutzstaffel (Elite Guards), or SS, as representative of the super Aryan race. Volunteer maidens were provided living quarters, a comfortable but not luxurious living, and medical attention. But this was a benign game compared to what followed.

Euthanasia would speed up cleansing of the race. A program to dispose of the unwanted was put underway by Kriminalkommissar **Wirth**. On the orders of the Reich Defense Council, the insane, feeble minded, and epileptic patients in hospitals, as well as residents of old age homes, were taken to institutions that specialized in killing them and cremating their bodies. Most of them were Germans but included also were hundreds of Poles and Russians. Relatives were not informed until after it happened, even if they had kept the patients hospitalized at their own cost. Most of them were told weeks later that the patient had died of an illness and that to prevent spread of an infection the body had to be cremated.

The clergy strongly opposed the practice, notably the Bishop of the Wuerttemberg Evangelical Provincial Church who wrote strongly worded letters of complaint to Reich Minister of the Interior **Wilhelm Frick**. There was no response. The supervisor at the sanatorium at Stettin and the Bishop of Limburg also wrote of their disapproval to the Reich Minister of Justice, but to no avail. There was no letup in eliminating people considered to be "useless eaters."

Even this systemized disposal of unwanted people by euthanasia was no match for the inhumane medical "experiments" conducted by Nazi doctors on concentration camp victims during the Holocaust. The purpose of the concentration camps was at first as slave labor camps. Anyone incapable of doing the work was simply exterminated ruthlessly, regardless of the reason for their incapacity. Old men and women, children, and cripples—all went to the gas chambers.[1]

The worst of the horror camps was Auschwitz where the commandant of the biggest mass murder in history was **Rudolf Hoess**. He was called for a conference in Berlin with **Heinich Himmler** who told him that the decision had been made at the highest level to exterminate the Jews as the only way to maintain the racial integrity of the German people.

The Nazi doctors used the abundant supply of prisoners to perform a staggering array of cold-blooded experiments on men, women, and children. The doctors claimed that their victims were volunteers because they knew that they would be killed anyway. Some had limbs amputated to see how they would make out, or to study their bones as if they were cadavers. Some were injected with chemicals such as phenol to see how long it would take them to die. Children were injected with gasoline. Some prisoners were put in a decompression chamber, and the air was pumped out. When the victims passed out they were removed and dissected while alive to determine the effect on their lungs.[2]

At the end of World War II the City of Nuremberg, Germany, was occupied by U.S. forces and held as part of the American zone. It was the site of the "Nuremberg Trials." War time President **Franklin D. Roosevelt** died April 12, 1945. The new president, **Harry Truman**, appointed Supreme Court Justice **Robert H. Jackson** to head the U.S. prosecution at the first of the Nuremberg trials in which Nazi officials were accused of crimes against international law. **Thomas J. Dodd** was named as the number 2 member of the prosecution team to serve as Justice Jackson's executive trial council. Dodd later became a U.S. representative, then a senator from Connecticut. His son, **Christopher J. Dodd** also became a senator from Connecticut.

Top Nazis were the first to be tried. Hitler's number 2 Nazi, **Herman Göring** (1893-1946) was sentenced to death by hanging, but the night before he was scheduled to be executed he committed suicide in his cell with hidden poison. Of the others: 11 were sentenced to death by hanging,

3 were sentenced to life in prison, 2 were sentenced to prison for 20 years, 1 was sentenced to prison for 10 years, 3 were found not guilty. **Rudolph Hess**, who was sentenced to life in prison, managed to commit suicide 41 years after the judgement of the tribunal. Thus, five of the top Nazis managed to escape by taking their own lives: Hitler, Göring, Hess, Himmler, and Goebbels.

There were thirteen trials in all, of which one was a trial of doctors who had conducted cruel medical experiments on people in concentration camps. The prosecutor, **Telford Taylor**, said in his opening statement,"… the twenty physicians in the dock range from leaders of German scientific medicine…down to the dregs of the German medical profession."[3]

Four of the Nazi doctors were hanged, and eight went to prison. The remaining defendants, as well as other suspects who were not tried, were allowed to return to their practices or affiliations.[4]

The lead doctor at Auschwitz, **Josef Mengele** (1911-1979), was a fanatic persecutor of Jews both before and during the war, and a cold blooded experimenter devoid of mercy for the victims. In one of his senseless experiments he injected more than a hundred pairs of twins with typhoid and tuberculosis bacteria, and after they died sent their organs to other scientists. Mengele, known as "Angel of Death" was at the Auschwitz extermination camp during 1943-45 where he directed the operation of the gas chambers and conducted his pseudoscientific racial studies. As a young man he had enlisted in the Sturmabteilung (Assault Division), and joined the research staff of the Institute for Hereditary Biology and Racial Hygiene. He served as a medical officer in the Waffen SS and in 1943 was appointed by **Heinrich Himmler** to be chief doctor at Birkenau, an extermination camp near Auschwitz. Mengele and his staff selected Jews for either labor or extermination, and he led experiments on inmates in an effort to find ways to increase fertility that could increase the quality of the German race. His chief interest was in research on twins. It's not clear how he escaped the Nuremberg trials. In 1949 he managed to get to South America, reportedly via Geneva, and settled in Uruguay as Jose Mengele, then to Paraguay where he was given citizenship. He died at a place near Sao Paulo, Brazil, never having been brought to justice.

CHAPTER 31

GOOD FROM EVIL

Can good come from evil? This is a true story of how it happened. The evil was a diabolical episode during WWII. Though only one of many atrocities committed during the war, the one we deal with here led to a scientific study that revealed the role that genetics could play in a disastrous circumstance. It expanded crucial information about the new science called *epigenetics*, revealing a new understanding of the nature/nurture relationship and how experiences can affect the health and welfare of people.

Background: WWII began September 1, 1939, when the Nazis attacked Poland using the German High Command's invention of warfare called *blitzkrieg* (lightning war) in which they attacked fortifications, industries, and troops using *Stuka* dive bombers, heavy bombers, tanks, and infantry. A month earlier Hitler and Stalin had made a secret agreement to take Poland and share it. On September 17, Russia also invaded Poland which surrendered on September 27, and the two aggressors split the country east and west.

The Germans turned west and quickly occupied Denmark, Norway, France and Romania, as well as sending a panzer unit to North Africa. In an effort to soften Britain for their intended invasion they battered London with their *Luftwaffe* (air force). Hitler announced that Germany would occupy the British Isles in one month, prompting Britain's Prime Minister **Winston Churchill** to make his historic declaration that he could offer the people nothing but "blood, toil, tears, and sweat."

The United States remained officially neutral but supported the British by giving England a fleet of forty "over-age" destroyers under a lend-lease agreement, and shipped other supplies to both England and France.

Germany countered with a fleet of U-boats (submarines) that sank many of the allied freighters with their torpedoes.

Neutrality ended when the Japanese attacked Pearl Harbor on December 7, 1941, with about 300 carrier-based planes, sinking three battleships, a mine layer and target ship and destroying at least 174 American planes. The same day, Japan declared war on the United States and Great Britain, and on the following day president **Franklin D. Roosevelt** signed a Congressional declaration of war. Roosevelt and Churchill met and agreed on a strategy of "beat Germany first." When allied forces stormed ashore at the Normandy beachhead on June 6, 1944, the stage was set for the advance on Germany.

Meanwhile, Germany invaded the Netherlands, forcing surrender in four days. The Netherlands, which had remained strictly neutral throughout World War I, did not take kindly to this incursion on their freedom. The Dutch people mounted an underground resistance to thwart the German occupation. Hitler retaliated by flooding all the ponders and establishing a rigid embargo. Shortage of food threatened the Dutch with starvation, and rationing only tended to equalize the agony of unrelenting hunger.

Remembered as the "Dutch Hunger Winter," the famine lasted for seven months in the winter of 1944-45 during which Dutch officials kept detailed documentation of health care records and food rationing.[1]

Bastiaan T. Heijmans, a molecular epidemiologist at the Leiden University Medical Center, and colleagues there and at Emory University, Columbia University, and New York State Psychiatric Institute, thought that any survivors of the Hunger Winter still alive, now 60 years or older, who were fetuses in their hungry mothers' wombs during the famine might carry in their cells a molecular record of the conditions. It is known that chemical changes in the DNA, described as *DNA methylation*, takes control of gene expression. The purpose of the study was to explore the possibility that mothers' diets may have been deficient in folate or other vitamins that provide the methyl moiety. Methylation is a principal modification in gene expression, that is, whether the gene will be expressed as originally programmed or whether it will remain silent. The effect is the same as a mutation except that the sequence in the gene makeup is the same as before the change in methylation.[2,3]

Richard Dawkins, a British biologist, in his 1976 book *The Selfish Gene* popularized the idea that genes vie with one another to be represented in the next generation, as if they are potentates at war to take over the domination of their subjects. Partly due to studies of the Dutch Hunger Winter, the gene is no longer thought of as the big enchilada. Contrary to the long-held view of its unassailable dominant role in determining anatomy and physiology of an organism, the findings of epigenetics reveal that the way a gene is, or is not, expressed is subject to modification and control. **Moshe Szyf**, an epigenetics researcher at McGill University in Montreal, was quoted, "It's all chemistry. What is most provocative here is the realization that the social environment can affect methylation." Methylation stops genetic expression without changing the DNA.

Many years later, using the Dutch workers' records, the investigators were able to locate nearly 1000 living adults who would have been fetuses about the time of the Dutch Hunger Winter. By drawing their blood and looking at the IGF2 gene, the gene involved in human growth and development, the scientists found 5% less DNA methylation than in people of an age that would not have made them fetuses during the Hunger Winter. Researchers found that children in the early stages of gestation were particularly vulnerable. Those exposed to famine later in development had lower birth rate but did not have the lower methylation. Dr. B.T.Heijmans: "Epigenetics could be a mechanism which allows an individual to adapt rapidly to changed circumstances. Changes in the DNA sequence occur by chance and it takes generations before a favourable mutation spreads throughout the population. By then a temporary famine is long past. It could be that the metabolism of children of the Hunger Winter has been set at a more economic level, driven by epigenetic changes." Children of the Hunger Winter are found to suffer more frequently from obesity which may be a result of this genetic change which allowed them to become more efficient at storing calories. Animal studies also show that the diet of mother mice affects differences in size, weight, and color of genetically identical offspring.

Randy L. Jirtle of Duke University who, with other epigenetic researchers, believes that genes in themselves are overly credited with explaining the biological framework. Jirtle was quoted, "Epigenetics is like the software that runs the genetic hardware." Then what, actually, is the genetic hardware and software? The word "epigenetics" was proposed by **C.H. Waddington** in the 1940s. A working definition of epigenetics (epi-*above*-genetics) is that it includes any system for the inheritance of traits that do not involve an alteration in the basic DNA code of the organism. In short, the inheritance of a variation in phenotype above and beyond the genome (DNA sequence) can be called epigenetic. Cells of multicellular organisms that contain genetic instructions all have the same DNA framework which one can say is the genetic hardware, inherited in a fixed pattern. But the DNA's performance can be modified by a chemically bound moiety stuck onto the DNA, figuratively, like a leach that can push or pull the influence of the DNA one way or another. Such is the action of methyl groups, which in number determine the degree of methylation and the effect on the size, shape, physiology, or performance of the organism. There is an effort to determine if a drug can be found that will reverse the abnormal epigenetic condition in cancers, such as blocking DNA methylation.[4]

It gives us a new way to appraise the old argument of the relative importance of nature versus nurture. Nurture has moved up a notch in our understanding of its influence on human health and welfare.[5, 6, 7]

CHAPTER 32

THE BARGAIN

On the other side of the globe no less heinous atrocities were being committed on prisoners in the guise of medical research on biological warfare (BW) agents. An investigation in depth by historian **Sheldon Harris** described what he called "death factories".[1] In an astonishingly low key development, much of it still shrouded in mystery, United States representatives covered up the horrors of medical "research" on humans and made a Faustian bargain with the Japanese BW scientists in return for purported "information" about their experiments. The culprits were allowed to avoid execution or other accountability for their crimes and to pursue their professional activities unpunished.

BACKGROUND: WAR WITH JAPAN
Early on the morning of December 7, 1941, a day described by president **Franklin D. Roosevelt** as "A Day of Infamy," Japanese carrier planes made a surprise attack on the Pearl Harbor Naval Base on the Hawaiian Island of Oahu.[2] One of the largest and best sheltered anchorages in the world, Pearl Harbor had 94 naval vessels, including eight battleships there at the time of the attack. Japan had amassed a striking force of 33 ships under the command of Vice Adm. **Chuichi Nagumo**, and under the cover of darkness approached to within 200 miles of the north coast of Oahu where the carriers launched about 360 airplanes, sinking three battleships and a minelayer as well as sinking or severely damaging 12 more ships. They also destroyed 170 American planes, most of them on the ground before they could take off, and afflicted about 3,700 casualties. "Remember Pearl Harbor!" became an American rallying call during the war.

On the same day, Japan attacked U.S. bases on Guam, Midway, Wake, and the Philippine capital of Manila. Two days later Japanese troops landed on Luzon where by December 22 there were more than 56,000 Japanese troops under the command of **Lt. General Masaharu Homma**. U.S. forces under **General Douglas MacArthur** withdrew to the rocky fortress of Corregidor in Manila Bay. President Franklin D. Roosevelt ordered MacArthur to be spirited away by torpedo boat, at which time the general made a famous pronouncement, "I shall return." **Lt. Gen. Jonathan M. Wainwright** was left in command of the 11,000 troop garrison. A shortage of food, ammunition, and medical supplies forced the garrison to surrender on May 6. Japanese soldiers showed no mercy. They forced 40,000 American and Philippine prisoners to march 70 miles over difficult tropical terrain to prison camps in what is known as the "Bataan Death March." Thousands of American and Philippine prisoners died from starvation, dehydration, exhaustion, injuries, and brutality.

The oldest survivor of the Bataan Death March died at the age of 105, August 14, 2011. **Albert Brown**'s story is told by author **Kevin Moore** in *Forsaken Heroes of the Pacific War: One Man's True Story*.[3] "Doc" Brown was 40, leaving behind a wife, children and a thriving dental practice when he was taken along with 78,000 prisoners, of whom 11,000 died, on the 65 mile march to a Japanese POW camp. He secretly made notes of the ordeal with a pencil stub and a tiny tablet hidden in the lining of a canvas bag. He told how they were denied food, water, and medicines. Those who stumbled or fell back were stabbed, shot, or beheaded. When the war ended in 1945, Brown was down to 100 pounds, having lost 80 pounds. He was nearly blind, recovering from a broken back and neck, and several diseases including malaria, dengue fever, and dysentery. He took two years to mend and for about 15 years could not bring himself to talk about his ordeal.

Early in 1942, a fleet of 16 B-25 army bombers under the command of Lt. Col. **James H. Doolittle** made a daring raid on the heartland of Japan. On April 18, they took off from the carrier *Hornet* and dropped bombs on Tokyo and other cities. The B-25s did not carry enough fuel to return to an allied base or any of the anticipated bases in China, so the pilots had to make out on their own. Doolittle and 63 of his fliers escaped with the help of the Chinese underground. One plane landed in Siberia. Eight fliers had to ditch, were caught by the Japanese and executed. The daring and bravery of Doolittle and his heroic fliers was a morale booster for the American public and gave the Japanese a shock because they didn't think enemy planes could ever reach them. Gen **Carl Spaatz**, in command of the U.S. Army Strategic Air Forces in the Pacific, and Maj. Gen. **Curtis E. LeMay**, in command of a fleet of B-29s, pulverized Tokyo and other cities with incendiaries and explosive bombs.

Kwajalein, which lies in the Marshall Islands, is the world's largest coral atoll. It was one of the "unsinkable carriers" taken from the Japanese as part of the island-hopping campaign devised by Adm. **Chester W. Nimitz**, in command of the Pacific Fleet, to bypass rather than attack many of the Japanese island bases. Early Japanese successes in which their carriers and *kamikaze* (suicide) dive bombers inflicted severe damage made it appear that Japan expected the allies to seek peace, but the outcome of subsequent naval and air battles turned the tide of the war. Land, sea, and air forces were brought to bear in the island-hopping campaign. Marines and army troops encountered fierce fighting on the beaches against stubborn defenders. Saipan was taken after suffering 14,000 U.S. casualties and killing 28,000 enemy soldiers.

On October 20, 1944, U.S. Army forces returned to the Philippines with a landing on the central island of Leyte, facing a 270,000-man Japanese army and a sizable air force. Five hours after the first landing Gen. MacArthur waded ashore, keeping his promise to return. The battle of Leyte Gulf was the biggest naval engagement in history and a decisive victory for the United States. Japan lost 4 carriers, 3 battleships, 10 cruisers, and 9 destroyers, almost the entire Japanese fleet. Desperation attacks by *kamikaze* (suicide) planes caused damage and casualties but were not decisive.

By July, 1945, Japan's war effort was in shambles. Its navy was destroyed and airplanes were too few to mount a defense. Nothing was left but ground forces. On July 26, the United States, Great Britain, and China demanded an unconditional surrender. Word came through Stalin that Japan would be willing to accept peace but not an unconditional surrender. The U.S. High command was convinced that to take control of Japan by a planned invasion of the Japanese home islands would be enormously costly in casualties, perhaps hundreds of thousands of lives. It was decided to use the atom bomb.[4]

In the early morning hours of August 6, 1945, on the Pacific island of Tinian, Pilot **Paul Tibbets** and his crew of a B-29 bomber, named the

Enola Gay, were ready to take off on a flight that would change the world forever. Within hours they were over the Japanese city of Hiroshima where they dropped "Little Boy," a uranium-based bomb. More than 70,000 people died and about as many were injured from the blast, radiation, or both. On August 9 a more powerful bomb, "Fat Boy," containing plutonium instead of uranium, was dropped on Nagasaki. It killed about 36,000 people and injured 40,000.

When President Truman announced that the Japanese had accepted Allied surrender terms on August 14, 1945, he named General **Douglas MacArthur** supreme commander of the Allied Powers. After officially accepting the surrender on the battleship U.S.S., Missouri, MacArthur set up headquarters in Tokyo and became sole administrator of the military-dominated government of Japan. One of the goals was to create a democratic government. Emperor **Hirohito** would be allowed to retain his crown but MacArthur ruled that the position would be purely ceremonial and that Hirohito would have no say in the government. The allies tried 28 of the top Japanese leaders for war crimes in which the Prime Minister, **Hideki Tojo**, and six others were executed. The other 21 were sent to prison. Pursuit of medical criminals involved in cruel and inhumane treatment of prisoners was astonishingly benign, notable for actually bargaining for immunity in return for information on their experiments with biological and chemical warfare agents.

On August 8, 1945, two days after Hiroshima was demolished by Little Boy, Russia declared war on Japan. Soviet troops advanced on the Siberia-Manchuria border for the immediate purpose of liberating Manchuria from Japanese control. A surprise finding was the remains of a vast network of testing establishments—for experiments in biological warfare (BW)—scattered along the edge of southwest China. The Japanese had destroyed them except those that were too large to obliterate in their hasty retreat. They were the sites of what investigator **Sheldon Harris** called "factories of death" that had been constructed in a way not obvious to the native residents who were not already imprisoned in them.[5]

In grim humor, victims were called *maruta* (logs of wood), probably referring to the practice of secretly burning used human and animal bodies instead of burying them, which would alarm residents. The maruta had to be destroyed quickly during the Japanese retreat. At one death factory on the outskirts of a town near the Russia-China border, the Soviet troops found a shallow grave containing at least 10,000 bodies—mostly Chinese and Mongolian men, women, and children. Some of them were still warm when the Soviets arrived.[6]

Japan had troops stationed in the Chinese province of Manchuria as early as 1905 to guard the South Manchurian Railway. When the Chinese began to strengthen their hold on Manchuria, a bombing "incident" on September 18, 1931, said to have been set off by Japanese troops, created the incentive for Japan to occupy all of Manchuria. They set up a puppet government and renamed the province Manchukua. Some historians say it was the start of WWII.

The civilian population of Manchuria and those near the southeastern border of occupied China, along with captured Korean and Chinese soldiers, as well as a few Russian and American POWs, provided abundant fodder for the Japanese military medical establishment to pursue experiments on biological warfare (BW). Selected victims were forced to submit to innumerable kinds of "experiments" by Japanese doctors.

An American POW who became a victim of experiments magically survived. **Lou Zamperini**, a B-24 bombardier told his story in a 2003 book, *Devil at My Heels* and a film made about him, *Still Carrying the Torch*. When his plane was shot down, he and two crew mates shared a raft that was strafed with 48 bullet holes that had to be painstakingly repaired while they were desperately trying to stay afloat. After drifting in sloshing water surrounded by sharks for 47 days during which the tail gunner died, they were captured by the Japanese and spent two years in POW camps. The worst was on Kwajalein where nine U.S. marines were executed and his captors turned him into, as Zamperini puts it, "a human guinea pig," injecting him with an array of mysterious drugs. He said that he and his fellow prisoners didn't worry because "We knew we were next, and if I die from these injections, that's better than having my head chopped off." He was rescued when the Japanese surrendered. Because he had been declared dead, his American rescuers at first refused to give him food or clothing. Fortunately, he had been able to retain his silver coliseum pass from his days as a USC athlete. As a track star he set the collegiate record in the mile that lasted for 15 years and led to participating in the 1936 Olympics in Berlin where he roomed with track star **Jesse Owens**.

Back home he married but fell into a life of addiction to alcohol, "...an alcoholic, chain smoker, rotten lowdown stinker." He was rescued from depravity by a meeting he attended where evangelist **Billy Graham** inspired him to change his life. Zamperini became an inspirational speaker himself with many affiliations and numerous commendations from civic groups.[7]

The mastermind of the Japanese biological and chemical warfare program was **Shiro Ishii**, an army medical officer who through exceptional energy, ambition, and accomplishments in biological warfare studies, achieved the rank of Lt. General.

Ishii's remarkable energy and sturdy constitution enabled him to handle his official duties with ease and aplomb. His quick mind and ingratiating demeanor enabled him to gain the support of senior medical officers for his plan to organize and supervise a network of facilities engaged in research on his favorite project: research and development of biological warfare agents.

Under Ishii's supervision 11 major BW research stations were established, mostly along the Manchurian border, where he and his fellow scientists would find an ample supply of human subjects for experiments among Chinese, Russian, and allied prisoners as well as hand-picked civilian villagers.[8]

Maj. General **Alden Waitt**, chief of the Chemical Corp at Fort Detrick, Maryland, the major facility of the U.S. Army Chemical Warfare Service (CWS), sent a parade of scientists to Tokyo to investigate vague reports of Japanese BW experiments.[9] The first was Lt. Col. **Murray Sanders**, a microbiologist who had worked on Japanese "B" encephalitis. His interpreter was English-speaking Lt. Col. **Naito Ryoichi** who, unknown to the Americans was a high ranking officer in the BW experiments. Next was Lt. Col. **Arvo T. Thompson**, a veterinarian well informed on BW research. He had the advantage of being the first to interview the Japanese BW top gun, General Shiro **Ishii**. Finally, General Waitt sent **Norbert H. Fell**, division chief of the Pilot-Engineering Section, a microbiologist with a Ph.D. from the University of Chicago, noted for his work on infectious diseases.

The Fort Detrick representatives told the Japanese they interviewed that they were not interested in looking for war crimes but for scientific information related to experiments on BW. The Japanese were not inclined to reveal information that might be used to incriminate them. They repeatedly lied, saying they knew nothing of such experiments. But investigations by intelligence officers in MacArthur's command uncovered convincing evidence of extensive BW research. They learned of the headquarters called Unit 731, the identity of some of the high ranking officers involved, and some of the BW research locations in China and Manchuria. The Japanese finally admitted that BW experiments had been conducted but declared that all records had been destroyed.

When Norbert Fell came on the scene, the statements were still devious, deceptive or contradictory. Ishii first said that he didn't know about any BW experiments, or couldn't remember, then bragged that he was in complete charge of the work at the headquarters station at Ping Fan and the main research unit 731. He told Fell that complete information would be given if he were provided with documentary proof that he, his subordinates and superiors would be given immunity.

Maj. General Waitt, in discussions with General MacArthur and other military personnel in Tokyo, argued that knowledge of the results of the Japanese atrocities was so vital in supplementing their work at Fort Detrick that it should be held in intelligence channels, kept secret, and not considered as war crimes. The American investigator **Sheldon H. Harris** contended that the data furnished by Ishii and others was of such minor significance that the cost in honor and integrity was high in comparison to the worth of the material obtained.[10]

Ishii and his BW experts involved in experiments on human victims were never charged with accountability as war criminals. Who decided, and when, that the Japanese BW criminals would be immune to war crimes prosecution? It was the opinion of Sheldon Harris that such a decision would have to be made at the highest level in Washington. The **Joint Chiefs**, president **Harry S. Truman**, his newly appointed secretary of defense **James Forrestal**, Gen. **George C. Marshall**, secretary of state, or one of their close subordinates, were theoretically the only ones qualified to authorize such action.[11]

The tortured mind of Forrestal may have been related to this episode. **James Vincent Forrestal** (1892-1949) was a navy aviator in WWI. He served as secretary of the Navy from 1944 to 1947 during which he helped build the United States fleet into the largest in the world. When in 1947 Congress unified the armed forces, President **Harry S. Truman** appointed Forrestal to be the first United States secretary of national defense. He resigned in 1949 and his suicide two months later was attributed by an unknown spokesman to stress from overwork and physical exhaustion. In

1954 the Navy named an aircraft carrier of a new class, the *Forrestal*, in honor of him.[12]

Benefits, if any, to the security of the United States from BW experiments of Lt. Gen. Shiro Ishii and his minions have not been revealed.

Following the surrender of Germany at the end of the European phase of World War II, trials were held at Nuremberg under the auspices of the United States representing the allies who were determined to bring to justice those responsible for the insufferable Nazi atrocities before and during the war. Unknown at the time to most people was that equally despicable atrocities were being conducted on the other side of the globe by people who were equally insensitive to the suffering of their victims.

It was 75 years ago that the people of Nanking, the ancient capital of China, were victimized by one of the worst atrocities in history, known as the Rape of Nanking. On December 13, 1937, the Japanese Imperial Army occupied Nanking during which thousands of women were forced to perform as sex slaves, called by the Japanese, "comfort women." An Allied investigation put the toll at more than 200,000 defenders killed and at least 20,000 women and girls raped during the six weeks after the city fell.

Investigators Bill Guttentag and Dan Sherman were impressed by the lack of remorse by the Japanese, even today. Guttentag is a lecturer at the Stanford Graduate School of Business and Dan Sherman was director of the Documentary film "Nanking" that won a Peabody Award in 2009. Guttentag and Sherman traveled to China and Japan to interview victims and soldiers who took part in the atrocity. One soldier, without a word of regret, told how they all drew straws, and the one who drew "first," proceeded to rape her. "We would take one girl and five of us would hold her down." A 79-year-old man told how as a nine year old he watched a soldier bayonet his mother to death as she breast fed his brother. Another man saw his 13-year-old sister sliced in half by a Japanese soldier because she resisted being raped. Elderly women told of rapes they endured as young girls.

The mass rapes of Nanking and the brutalization of the people finally convinced the Japanese military leaders that they would have to bring things under control. They had soldiers round up women and force them to serve as sex slaves in what the Japanese called "comfort stations". Japan's election (in 2012) of the ultraconservative nationalistic **Shinzo Abe** as prime minister was seen by many Chinese as a continuation of insults. For example, Japan's proposal to nullify a 1993 apology for the thousands of women the Japanese army sexually enslaved during World War II. Under prime minister Abe there followed a series of denials, and distortions of the truth, mainly that they were propaganda spread by China. A professor at a Japanese university insisted that there were no killings or rapes in Nanking. Another argument was that Franklin D. Roosevelt had forced Japan to go to war in an effort to lift the U.S. out of the depression, or simply that the U.S. forced Japan into bombing Pearl Harbor.[13]

PART VII
MICE

33 Of Mice And Medicine

34 Human Mice And The Gulf War

CHAPTER 33

OF MICE AND MEDICINE

Jackson Laboratory, a nonprofit organization in Bar Harbor, Maine, makes a specialty of breeding mice with specific genetic characteristics, such as susceptibility to a particular disease or human ailment. The laboratory's strains cover a wide spectrum of disorders from Alzheimer's to arthritis. Sequencing both human and mouse genomes reveals that we are remarkably similar in genetic makeup, consequently similar in physiology. Differences often involve when, where, and how genes are activated. The Jackson lab offers more then 5,000 strains of mice. The most popular strain is the "Black 6" developed in 1921, used to study a wide variety of disorders from diabetes to obesity. Some of the Black 6 mice even took a trip in the space shuttle. During one year (2007) Jackson supplied 2.4 million mice to 16,000 researchers worldwide.[1]

The Jackson Laboratory (also called Jax), was founded in Bar Harbor, Maine, in 1929 by **Clarence Cook Little**, former president of University of Maine and University of Michigan. It was named the Roscoe B. Jackson Memorial Laboratory.

The Jackson Laboratory is an independent, non-profit biomedical research institute. Its mission is to discover the genetic basis for preventing, treating, and curing human diseases. It is the world-wide source of genetically defined mice. Mice and humans share 95% of their genes, so mice are an efficient model for human diseases. Jackson Laboratory is the home of the mouse genome database and an international hub for scientific courses, conferences, training, and education. At least 22 Nobel prizes were associated with Jackson Laboratory research, mouse models, and educational programs. The facility at Sacramento, California, was established to accommodate researchers on the West Coast.[2]

A common figure of speech when referring to experiments on people is "human guinea pigs." Books have been written on it, and endless talk is concerned with the ethics of it. But guinea pigs, while still used for experimentation, lost favor to the more prolific and easily managed rats as substitutes for the study of human physiology and of reactions to germs and drugs. Ferrets are sometimes used, such as for flu studies. But the most favored of all are mice, especially for physiology and genetic studies.

Although large animals of several kinds are used for some studies, the most useful in final evaluations of new medicines are humans. It would have meaning to say that people used for such experiments are *human mice*. If you ever used prescription drugs, or anything stronger than a tried and true remedy such as aspirin, it's almost certain that you participated indirectly in experiments on people. It's generally agreed that experiments on humans is an essential step in developing a new drug. Whenever we buy a prescription medicine or almost any over-the-counter drug, we are buying one that was approved, if in the United States, by the U.S. Food and Drug Administration (FDA), hopefully only after experiments on humans to determine its safety and effectiveness.

They are not called experiments. They are called clinical trials. Hundreds of clinical trials are in progress, most of them presumably conducted ethically and in the best interests of the human participants. But not always. And not all experiments were for evaluation of medicines. Some experiments of the recent past in the United States and elsewhere were flagrant violations of human decency. A physician, **M. Prinzmetal**, wrote in 1965, "During my training in medical school, as well as my residency in St. Louis, fellowships at Harvard, New York City, and London, and visits to Vienna, Budapest, and other European medical centers, I was always horrified by the inhumane manner in which charity patients were treated."[3] But none can compare with the reprehensible treatment of Jews and others in concentration camps by Nazi doctors during the Holocaust, and equally despicable use of conscripted Chinese and other captives in a campaign to test biological weapons by the Japanese.

Guidelines and ethical standards for trials on humans are clearly defined. The most important requirement is *informed consent*. Unfortunately, there's an unintended fudge factor making the "informed" part of the rule flexible, the amount and kind of information being given to the participants usually being determined by those conducting the trial. Voluntary "consent" can be under a cloud of uncertainty. Can small children give informed consent? No. But parental consent is accepted. Is the consent of prisoners who are offered leniency, or who simply expect favorable treatment, true voluntary consent? To what extent can patients in mental hospitals give informed consent? In numerous cases consent is not specifically asked for, nor is much information given. Many trials are conducted by contractors who find it economically advantageous to get the information by outsourcing their work in backwater locations in foreign lands where the people are poor and not apt to understand much about the purpose of the trial.

Much of the early work on humans initiated by medical staffs were clumsy, poorly planned, grossly insensitive experiments that yielded little useful information, and more often than not, leaving the victims to suffer from adverse effects. In the United States, some experimental work in psychosurgery appears to have been racially motivated. Experiments were conducted at the University of Mississippi in Jackson on emotionally distressed and abandoned African-American children. The director of neurosurgery, **O. J. Andy**, would insert multiple electrodes into the brains of children as young as five. Experiments would sometimes be repeated several times over periods of months or years to determine the outcome in older children or even adults. At about the same time, Harvard Medical School's neurosurgeons **Vernon Mark** and **William Street** implanted dozens of electrodes in the brains of patients on the theory that it would curb violence. They theorized that black urban rioters had a disease that could be cured by brain surgery.[4]

A notorious case of human exploitation was the Tuskegee experiment, so-called because it enlisted male African-American sharecroppers living in an area near Tuskegee in Macon County, Alabama, where the rate of syphilis infection in the black community was exceptionally high. The "experiment," started in 1932 and lasting four decades, was the brain child of **Taliaferro Clark**, a physician with the Public Health Service (PHS). The concept was foggy at best. Instead of providing the best medical treatment available, the idea was to withhold therapeutic treatment to see how the disease progressed. Would it be different than in whites? Would the patients be just as well off without treatment? What would autopsies reveal?

About 400 men who said they were ill with "bad blood," actually syphilis, were recruited along with about 200 healthy men as controls. The government researchers asked the local doctors to refrain from treating the subjects of the study and with unabashed deception gave them regular "treatments" with mercury ointment, long known to be ineffective, as well as aspirin and tonics, and pampered them with free lunches, even burial insurance.

The Tuskegee researchers gave a report on their preliminary findings at the 1936 annual meeting of the American Medical Association (AMA). Their conclusion? The untreated sick patients were getting sicker than the controls. Although penicillin, a highly effective treatment for syphilis, became available in the early 1940s, it was withheld from the patients. The government doctors appealed to local draft boards to have the army refrain from the new treatment to preserve the "integrity" of the experiment.

The experiment ended in late 1972 after a former Public Health Service investigator, **Peter Buxton**, exposed the unethical procedures to an Associated Press reporter. By then 28 participants had reportedly died of syphilis, 100 died of related complications, at least 40 wives had been infected, and 19 children contracted the disease at birth.[5] Public knowledge of the experiment prompted heated debates among doctors, scientists, public officials, and legislators that ultimately led to ethical guidelines for experiments on humans, the foremost of which are full disclosure of the purpose and procedures, and permission by the participants.

CHAPTER 34

HUMAN MICE AND THE GULF WAR

The Gulf War set the stage for an experiment, maybe the world's biggest, on the effect of chemicals on humans. The innovative use of a medicine given to American soldiers to protect them against the possibility of a nerve gas attack had unintended health effects. The symptoms suffered by veterans for years afterward were so severe, diverse, and widespread that the U.S. Congress mandated a thorough study of the cause or causes.

On August 2, 1990, Iraq invaded and quickly subdued the small but oil-rich country of Kuwait. **Saddam Hussein's** Iraq troops, accompanied by a horde of plundering civilians, seized everything of value they could find, including the oil fields and equipment. Intending to include Kuwait as part of Iraq, Hussein formally annexed the country on August 8. United States president **George H. W. Bush** (the first president Bush) saw the need to launch a rescue operation to counter Hussein's ambition of dominating the Mideast oil supply on which so many people throughout the world depended. He sent Secretary of State **James A. Baker**, a masterful negotiator, to all major countries that might be interested and obtained almost universal support for an invasion.

The United Nations Security Council (UN) called on Iraq to withdraw. Several European countries, along with Egypt and other Arab countries, rushed troops to the Saudi Arabian staging area. By January 15, allied strength had reached 700,000 troops including 540,000 U.S. troops and other personnel.

On January 16-17, 1991, under the planning and leadership of four-star general **Colin W. Powell**, chairman of the Joint Chiefs of Staff, the United States led with a massive air offensive in an operation called Desert Storm. On February 24, operation Desert Sabre was launched from Saudi Arabia into Kuwait and southern Iraq. The elite forces of Iraq tried to make a stand but were defeated. President Bush declared a cease fire on February 28. The allies lost about 300 soldiers; thousands of Iraqis were killed.

After the Gulf War, a worrisome number of veterans complained of puzzling health problems that defied both diagnosis and treatment. Some of the ailments were of disabling severity. For want of a better name it came to be known as the Gulf War Syndrome, affecting about a fourth of the U.S. troops who served in the conflict. Neurological symptoms ranged from fatigue, memory loss, concentration problems, rashes, and widespread pain. The veterans also had higher rates of brain cancer and amyotrophic lateral sclerosis (Lou Gehrig's disease). One study indicated that 26-32% of personnel deployed in the Gulf War developed chronic health problems.[1]

During years of complaints of debilitating ailments by veterans, many of them were turned down for treatment with the explanation that their troubles didn't exist, merely the result of wartime stress. The army was asked to make a thorough study of the cause. Much was made of the possibility that a unit had been affected by nerve gas during demolition of Iraq's Khamisiyah munitions depot. The DOD estimated that about 100,000 personnel may have been exposed to a low level of nerve gas Sarin. Several studies were made by the Institute of Medicine (IOM), an arm of the prestigious National Academy of Science. Their conclusion was the usual war-time medical suspect: "Psychological effects from the strains and stress of war and other unknown causes," sometimes referred to as post traumatic stress disorder (PTSD).

Veterans and their families, as well as many others, were not satisfied with the IOM inconclusive studies. The investigation seemed to be incomplete to many people. Barely mentioned in early public statements, and ignored in the IOM conclusion, was an obvious possibility: unintended effects of what was probably the most massive experiment ever conducted on humans.

Dr. Harold Cox, chairman of one of the IOM studies, and editor of *Annals of Internal Medicine*, was quoted, "There's something about going to the Gulf and serving in the Gulf that has caused something bad and persistent and real, but we have not found any evidence for a specific cause."

Members of Congress became increasingly concerned about the plight of the veterans. In 2002, Congress commissioned a "Research Advisory

Committee on Gulf Warfare Veterans' Illnesses" to further study the problem. Two-thirds of the 15-member panel were scientists. **Robert F. White**, associate dean of research at Boston University School of Public Health, who was the panel's scientific director, was quoted, "Some people feel that the IOM reports have been permission to ignore these guys." The panel asked Congress to appropriate $60 million a year for research on finding a cure. Their 450-page report was released in November 2008, and delivered to the Secretary of Veterans Affairs **James Peake** with the statement:

The extensive body of research now available indicates that Gulf War illness is real, that it is a result of neurotoxic exposures during Gulf War deployment, and that few veterans have recovered or substantially improved with time.

The panel cited two primary causes of the illnesses:

Overuse of the drug pyridostigmine bromide (PB).
Exposure to a wide variety of pesticides, often overused.[2,3]

At the outset of the Gulf War the troops were given pills intended to give protection against nerve gas poisoning. The active ingredient of the medicine, pyridostigmine bromine (PB), was already in use as the favored medical treatment for an ailment called *myasthenia gravis*, a rare condition caused by a malfunction of the same biochemical system that is the target of nerve gas poisoning.

PB must have been tested on volunteers, and if so, the results will probably remain secret. Admittedly, it had not been sufficiently tested to have FDA approval as a protection against nerve gas, but the army was given a waiver because the use of nerve gas by Iraq was seen as an imminent threat. PB pills were offered to all the troops. Officially, they were not required to take them but there was pressure to do it. Many of the troops said later that they were not told they had a choice. At least 250,000 troops took them. Records were not kept.

PB tablets when used as medicine to treat myasthenia gravis are provided either as conventional 60 milligram tablets or so-called Timespan 180 milligram tablets. The usual dose is ten 60 milligram tablets per day spaced to provide maximum relief. In severe cases as many as 25 tablets daily may be required. The dose for the Timespan tablets of 160 milligrams is one to three tablets taken once or twice a day or as needed.[4, 5] Since it would be inconceivable for the army to deploy troops sick with myasthenia gravis for on line duty, **any** dose of PB would be an **overdose**. Questioning personnel about how many PB pills they had taken led to the conclusion that those who took the most pills had worse symptoms than those who took fewer PB pills.

The discovery and development of PB has a colorful past. When in the 1700s-1800s Europeans discovered that Africa could provide valuable products for import to America, the West Indies, and other tropical areas of the New World, they established trading posts along the west coast of Africa. One of them was at a place called Old Calabar in a province of what is now Nigeria. There was a tribe called Efiks who were eager to provide items of value, especially palm oil and slaves. A settlement of Efiks had a chief who, along with a council of elders, made decisions on tribal affairs including strict punishment for anyone who violated standards of behavior, especially witchcraft. In order to determine guilt or innocence the accused was given an "ordeal poison," a soupy potion containing a small amount of water in a mixture with eight macerated dried seeds of a perennial woody climbing plant (named by botanists *Physostigma venenosum*) that grows on banks of streams in tropical West Africa. The Efiks called the seeds, as well as the ritual, *sere*. The Europeans dubbed them "calabar beans."

William Freeman Daniel, a medical officer in the British army, witnessed an ordeal trial in 1846 and wrote an account of it. The accused was required to swallow the slurry of calabar beans and ordered to walk around until the effect was evident. Then if the person could raise the right hand and vomit the poison, he or she was pronounced innocent. If not, the accused would die a horrible death.[6]

A theory is that the calabar bean may actually work to prove guilt or innocence. The supposition is that an innocent subject would not hesitate to promptly swallow the poison, resulting in nausea and regurgitation, whereas a guilty subject would most likely stall, chewing and swallowing slowly, hoping to defer any poisonous effect, actually guaranteeing a fatal result.[7]

In 1863 some of the calabar beans arrived at the botanic garden in Edinburgh, Scotland, where **Robert Christison**, a professor of medicine at the University of Edinburgh, tested the effect of the poison by ingesting a small amount of the bean. He survived. His assistant, **Thomas Fraser**, isolated the poisonous ingredient and named it *eserine*. A year later the pure alkaloid was identified and renamed *physostigmine*. Its first use as a medicine was by **L. Lacqueur** who in 1877 used it as a treatment for glaucoma.[8] When applied to the eye, physostigmine causes the pupil to constrict, in contrast to atropine which causes dilation.

Physostigmine has a chemical configuration described as a *carbamate*. That knowledge led to the synthesis of a variety of carbamates in a search for insecticides and medicines, of which PB is one.

A medicine that has been used for decades as an antidote for nerve gas and poisons of similar action is *atropine*, an alkaloid of the deadly nightshade, *Atropa belladona*, also in Jimpson weed, *Datura stramonium*. Its effectiveness and limitations are well known. But at the outset of the Gulf war the army decided that PB could be used as a prophylactic, that is, a preventive, not as an antidote, against nerve gas. It would be a dramatic innovation in treating nerve gas poisoning. The so-called nerve gases are the most heavily stockpiled chemical agents for modern warfare. They belong to a group of chemicals called *organophosphates*, such as Sarin, favored by the United States and Russia and easily manufactured by others.

The poisonous effect of an organophosphate nerve gas is to cause the uninterrupted presence of the neurotransmitter, acetylcholine, causing convulsions and probably a quick death.

Back to myasthenia gravis, in which the problem of the malady is not from too much acetylcholine (as in nerve gas poisoning) but lack of enough of it, which results in muscular weakness, in some cases extreme, and numerous related problems. So why not do something to get rid of actylcholine's nemesis, the enzyme acetylcholinesterase? One of the organophosphate insecticides, TEPP (Tetraethylpyrophosphate), was tested for that but it was too dangerous. What's needed is a medicine that acts in a similar way, only very much milder. An array of substances can do that. The medical profession selected PB, for myasthenia gravis, allowing an increase in the acetylcholine neurotransmitter needed in small amounts. By any standard, the carbamate PB is a weak poison compared to organophosphates such as Sarin. Why would a weak poison prevent the effects of a stronger one? Can a poison kill a poison?

In 1954, Canadian scientists **W. L. Ball**, **J. W. Sinclair**, **M. Crevier**, and **K. Kay** made a surprising discovery. They found that a single injection in rats of any of three chlorinated hydrocarbon insecticides that they tested gave marked protection against parathion, a highly poisonous organophosphate insecticide.[9] There was protection only if the chlorinated compounds were injected first, some time before application of the parathion. Using them in reverse order was ineffective. In 1958, German scientists, **D. Neubert,** and **J. Schaefer**[10] showed that a single injection in mice of a chlorinated hydrocarbon protected the mice from either paraoxon or Schradan (organophosphate poisons). Again, to be effective the protective agent had to be applied first, some time before the other poison. In 1964, scientists **R. M. Welch** and **J. M. Coon** found several compounds including phenobarbitol gave protection against organophosphates and pyridostigmine. In 1970, **W. K. Barry** and **D. R. Davies** reported that carbamates as well as atropine can be antidotes against organophosphate toxicants.[11] And **H. W. Dorough** reported the protective effect of a carbamate on the toxicity of methyl parathion to mice. Again, in all of these experiments effective protection depended on administering the carbamate before the organophosphate poison.[12, 13] There was no protection when used in reverse order.

As for how a poison would protect against another poison, **Richard D. O'Brien**, a toxicologist at Cornell University, states, "A...plausible explanation would be that liver-degrading enzymes were induced by the pretreatments."[14, 15] It is a logical assumption that may apply broadly to a wide range of protective poisons. (Dr. O'Brien was referring to the remarkable ability of the liver to manufacture detoxifying enzymes. A family of several dozen related enzymes called *cytochrome p450 enzymes* are always ready to attack dangerous or unwanted chemicals in the blood stream. They will modify the structure of the invader to make it nontoxic or render it more easily eliminated by the kidneys. Unlike most enzymes, cytochrome p450 enzymes are nonspecific. They make a wide variety of insoluble chemicals soluble by adding oxygen, thus enabling them to be flushed out. Adding oxygen can also be useful as with vitamin A and E which require it to be in an active form. Cytochrome p450 enzymes can be a problem with drugs (virtually all are poisons) by either rendering them useless or even making them dangerous. It's a reason for evaluating drugs thoroughly before using them.)[16]

Then there is the question about the effect of pesticides. At least 64 pesticides, containing 37 different active ingredients were sprayed around dining and living areas as well as on tents and uniforms. One possibility of a pesticide contributing to the Gulf War Syndrome was the use of an insect repellent, diethyl toluamide (DEET), applied to the skin or clothing. There may have been an unintentional interaction between two or more of the chemical ingredients. A common practice with some pesticides is to use them in mixture with a chemical known to produce a synergistic effect, that is, an enhanced effect greater than when used alone. It is not necessary for both chemicals in the mixture to be toxic but if the added chemical is also toxic, synergism will make the effect more than additive. Synergism may have been the case with PB. A study by a Department of Agriculture researcher, **James Moss**, found that DEET in mixture with PB was several times more active than when each was used alone.[17]

Still further complicating the puzzle of the Gulf War syndrome was that Hussein was suspected of having stockpiled both anthrax and botulinum weapons. About 150,000 of the troops were given at least one anthrax vaccination, and 8,000 were given at least one dose of botulism vaccine (BT). Knowledge of the long term effects of these vaccines is limited. Both anthrax vaccine and BT vaccine can have serious side effects. The BT used during the Desert Storm campaign was still "investigational" and in any case may have been ineffective. The material used was 20 years old and only two doses per person were given although four doses over a year's time were believed to be necessary.[18]

So what can we conclude about the cause of the Gulf War Syndrome? We have as facts an experiment in which thousands of *human mice* (soldiers) were given the drug *pyridostigmine bromide* (PB) already in use to treat patients sick with a disorder, called *myasthenia gravis*, in which the neurotransmitter hormone *acetylcholine* (ACh) is absent or extremely low. The remedial action of PB in treating myasthenia gravis is to block the natural enzyme *acetylcholinsterase* (AChE) that would normally destroy ACh, thus leaving ACh to transmit nerve impulses across the neuromuscular junctions throughout the central and peripheral nervous systems.

But the soldiers were not sick (yet). They did not need more Ach and they did not need medicinal PB except for the army's belief that its use could stimulate the physiological system to protect soldiers against a nerve gas attack. However, blocking AchE in a healthy person will cause an excess of ACh that can be damaging in a number of ways.

Excessive use of insecticides may have been another cause of Gulf War Syndrome but proof is hard to establish.

The congressional panel's chairman, **James H. Binns**, a former deputy assistant secretary of Defense and a Vietnam veteran was quoted, "The tragedy here is that there are no current treatments."

The question is, how many of the afflicted Gulf War veterans still surviving will live long enough to benefit from treatments, if ever found?

PART VIII
HEALING AND THE MIND

35 Fountain Of Youth

36 The Power Of Belief

37 Faith Healers

38 Mesmerism

39 Biofeedback

40 A Self Healer

CHAPTER 35

FOUNTAIN OF YOUTH

Everybody wants to live a long life but nobody wants to get old. Why do we grow old? Why does youth slip away, leaving us with crippling old age? Is living into the stratospheric years beyond the traditional four score and ten with unimpaired vigor an impossible achievement? People have pondered questions of aging since ancient times. According to the Old Testament book of Genesis, Methuselah, the grandfather of Noah, lived 969 years. Babylonians believed that some of their heroes lived 36,000 years.

Juan Ponce de Leon (1460-1521), a Spanish explorer, achieved everlasting fame for his search for the Fountain of Youth. He had been told by native American Indians in the Bahamas of a spring that would rejuvenate and give everlasting youthful life to anyone who drank from it. So he sampled every body of water that he encountered, testing the waters for the supposed Fountain of Youth.

Ponce de Leon was a page in the Royal court of Ferdinand of Aragon when Christopher Columbus discovered the New World. He may have begun his career of exploration as part of Columbus's second expedition. He served as the captain of a ship under the governor of the West Indies area of the Caribbean known as Hispaniola. He embarked on an expedition in 1513 and landed on the east coast of Florida which he presumed was an island. He named it Florida because of the lush vegetation and because it was discovered at Easter time. After sailing through the Keys to Florida's west coast he returned to Spain and was appointed military governor of Bimini and Florida with permission to colonize them. With two ships and 200 men he explored the coast west of Florida where at one landing they engaged in a fight with a band of Seminole Indians in which Ponce was badly wounded by an arrow. He was returned to the headquarters port in Cuba, where he died.

But the dream did not die. **James Hilton** fanned the flame with his 1933 book *Lost Horizon* in which four people stranded in Baskul during an uprising were offered a ride to safety in a private airplane designed to fly at high altitudes.[1] To their surprise, the pilot had been forcibly removed and the new pilot flew them in a direction different from what they expected. He made a crash landing high in the Tibet mountains. A lama appeared who guided them to his lamasery, Shangri-La, in a remote valley, an Eden-like garden with a clear sky and balmy climate. It was a utopian paradise where people lived years beyond the average human life span, and aged very slowly in appearance. A place where time seemed to stand still. The people of Shangri-La lived a life of moderation. There were no policemen because there was no crime. Everyone was moderately engaged in reading, writing, playing the harpsichord or piano, or leisurely tending crops in the irrigated low part of Shangri-La.

A movie was made of *Lost Horizon* in 1937, starring **Ronald Colman** and **Jane Wyatt**. It was wildly popular, shown repeatedly through the years. President **Franklin D. Roosevelt** (1882-1945) liked to call the presidential retreat at Camp David, Shangri-La. The legend drew travelers to where they imagined Shangri-La might be. A resort called Shangri-La is a popular tourist attraction. It was reported that a Nazi expedition led by **Ernst Schäfer** went to Tibet in 1938 hoping to find an ancient master race unspoiled by civilization.[2]

Scientists and pseudo-scientists did not ignore the search for everlasting youth. Questions of aging, its causes, and possible control stimulated a vast amount of theorizing and scientific investigations. Among the early searchers of the Fountain of Youth were those who thought they could rejuvenate men's sexual powers. **Brown-Séquard**, a French physician and professor at the University of Paris, at the age of 72 thought wistfully of his vanished youth and pondered ways that he might rejuvenate his flagging virility. Who, he thought, would be more capable of studying and evaluating an experiment of virility than a 72-year-old man with basic knowledge of physiology and experience in observing the effects of medical treatments? *Mais naturellement, le docteur* himself.

Dr. Brown-Séquard made extracts of guinea pig and dog testicles, injected them into himself and was convinced that it made him gain in vigor. In his report published in 1889 he described the benefits he experienced.[3] Unknown to Dr. Brown-Séquard or anyone else, his preparations must not have contained much of the chief male hormone because when testosterone is injected it is quickly changed in the cells to a form that is not soluble in water.[4] His results were probably mostly examples of the well-known placebo (an inert medicine) effect.

A company physician, whose name I will not disclose, described the powerful placebo effect on sexual performance. When giving annual physical examinations to male employees occasionally one would mention a sexual problem and ask, "Doc, can you do anything about it?" The doctor would invariably reply, "Sure I can," and would proceed to inject a small amount of sterile saline with the comment that it would last a long time (this was in the pre-Viagra days). Often the man would return later to thank the doctor for that wonderful medicine.

Brown-Séquard's experiments stimulated widespread and lasting interest in the magical effects of animal glands. Writer **Somerset Maugham** was one of many people who went to Switzerland for injections of goat hormones after which he lived into his 91st year with no complaints heard about his virility. The placebo effect has valuable use in the development of medicines (described in chapter 36) but it can be used also for fraudulent purposes. During the 1920s and early 1930s, **John R. Brinkley** established in the United States a thriving practice of supposedly transplanting goat testicles into aging men. He recruited patients by radio commercials. Brinkley held an M.D. degree from a diploma mill and some sort of honorary degree from the University of Pavia, Italy. He was licensed to practice medicine in several states.

"Doctor" Brinkley started a clinic in Milford, Kansas, where he soon became a millionaire charging a minimum of $750 (equivalent to at least twice today's money) for a "transplant." Glands of a very young goat would cost $1,500. The operation took twenty minutes. Brinkley's radio station license was revoked, so he moved to Mexico and set up a station across the Rio Grande from Del Rio, Texas. He pretended to perform prostate operations and sold a concoction made of very weak hydrochloric acid colored with a blue dye. He sported several cars and yachts and a private airplane in which he flew back and forth to a hospital he established in Little Rock, Arkansas. He was narrowly defeated in one of his three tries for governor of Kansas.

Several researchers experimented with implanting gonads of monkeys and apes. In 1929, **S. Voronoff** implanted ape testicles into aging men with what he claimed to be beneficial results.[5] The procedure was tried by believers in both Europe and the United States.

As for the effect of gonads on aging, a 1969 study of eunuchs in an institutional population of mentally retarded inmates was reported by **J. B. Hamilton** and **G. E. Mestler** who concluded that there was no difference in life span from normal individuals.[6]

More than 400 years after the Spanish explorer's futile effort to find the fountain of youth, scientific studies with laboratory rats indicated that there might, in fact, be a way to prolong youthful life. In 1935 a team of nutritionists, **C.M. McCay**, **M.F. Crowell**, and **L. A. Maynard** at Cornell University made a surprising discovery. They found that restricting the diet of young rats made them live longer.[7] There followed a series of studies by others that confirmed the finding of McCay and his associates. In a 1968 experiment **D.S. Miller** and **P. R. Payne** increased rats' length of life 28% by feeding them a high protein diet for the first four moths of their lives and after that a very low protein diet.[8] In 1974 **M. H. Ross** and **G. Bras** added to previous work by showing that the onset of age-related diseases can be controlled by the rat's diet.[9]

Could youthful life of people be prolonged the same way as with rats? There was not much enthusiasm. Who would want to experiment with humans the same way as with rats? The average life span of rats is about three years, making it easy to repeat or confirm findings. With people, results would have to wait decades for them to die to determine life span. By then, researchers themselves might be dead. Moreover, **Gairdner B. Moment** of the Department of Biological Sciences, Gouche College, Baltimore, who evaluated the effects of the diet regimes on the health of the rats, noted that some of the rats on restricted diets appeared sickly, others were sterile, still others while healthy were undersized as determined by researchers Miller and Payne.[10] The diets would have to be checked out on primates, and eventually on humans.

Despite questions, widespread interest in all aspects of aging continued. The U.S. Congress passed the Research on Aging Act of 1974, creating a National Institute on Aging under the National Institutes of Health, and the Gerontology Research Center in Baltimore together with the Adult Development and Aging Branch as parts of the National Institute of Child

Health and Human Development with oversight by a National Advisory Council on Aging.

Where does all this lead us to in the question of diet and life span of people? Believers in the possibility were encouraged by reports that animals and other organisms unrelated to rats or humans also lived longer if their caloric intake was restricted. Rats, mice, yeast, round worms, fish, and monkeys, all responded to reduced diet by prolonged life. Dietary restrictions of *Drosophila* flies increased their life span, reduced mortality rate, and drastically reduced female fecundity.[11]

There are some dedicated believers in extending their life span by diet restriction and control. **Paul McGlothin** and **Meredith Averill**, a married couple now in their early 60s have for more than 16 years been eating a carefully selected diet restricted in calories, as told by C&EN West Coast News Bureau representative **Laura Cassiday**, who interviewed the couple in 2009.[12] Cassiday says that the couple "….are often mistaken for being much younger than their years. They say they feel almost 20 years younger. Their blood pressure, resting heart rates, and body fat percentages rival those of Olympic athletes."

McGlothin and Averill belong to a group called the Calorie Restriction Society, a group of people who restrict their calorie intake, convinced that it will improve health and slow aging. They call themselves CRONies (Calorie Restriction with Optimal Nutrition). Cassiday reported that the group was studied by **Luigi Fontana**, an Associate Professor of medicine at Washington University School of Medicine in St. Louis and director of the Division of Nutrition and Aging at Instituto Superiore di Sanita, Rome, Italy. Cassiday quoted Fontana, "On the basis of their metabolic profile, CRONies have practically zero risk of developing cardiovascular disease or stroke….these people have hearts that are 15 years younger in terms of biology."

D. K. Ingram, **George Roth** and collaborators at the National Institute of Aging and **J. W. Kemnitz** and **Richard Weindruch** at the University of Wisconsin, Madison, made a 20-year study of calorie restriction in rhesus monkeys. Placed on calorie-restriction diets at 7 to 14 years-old, when they reached old age they appeared younger than the controls, had significantly reduced cases of diabetes, cancer, and cardiovascular disease. There was less age-related brain atrophy and muscle wasting. Control animals had a three-fold higher death rate from age-related causes. At the time of the report, the calorie-restricted monkeys had an 80% survival rate compared to 50% of the control animals. After 20 years in the trial the animals began to die from age-related causes. Early results indicate that those on restricted diets are outlasting their well-fed friends. The life span of rhesus monkeys is about 40 years. Time will tell whether that can be extended.[13, 14]

The first time a drug has shown an increase in longevity of an animal was when scientists tested a secretion of a dirt-dwelling bacterium from Easter Island on mice. The drug, called *rapamycin*, is prescribed by doctors to combat kidney cancer and to prevent rejection of transplanted organs. **David E. Harrison**, **Randy Strong**, and workers at the Jackson Laboratory in Bar Harbor, Maine, in collaboration with **Richard A. Miller**, a professor at the University of Michigan, fed rapamycin to mice when they were 600 days old, comparable to 60-year-old people, increasing mice longevity by 9% to 14%.[15] Rapamycin would not be a candidate for human use to increase life span because it impairs the immune system. Researchers hope that knowledge of its action on longevity might lead to something more promising.

Not surprisingly, recent studies by social psychologists **E. Diener** (Institute of Metabolic Sciences, University of Cambridge, Cambridge, UK) and **M.Y. Chan** (Department of Economics, University of Zurich, Switzerland) showed that happiness has a positive effect on physiological health and longevity. An analysis based on 24 studies using different methods gave an estimate that happy people live 14% longer than those who said they were unhappy. In a survey of people in industrial countries, happier people had an increased longevity of 7.5 to 10 years. The investigators also found that happier people are less apt to commit suicide and less likely to have accidents.[16]

CHAPTER 36

THE POWER OF BELIEF

The mind plays a role in health and healing, and a major part of the mind's involvement is *belief*—belief in something: a thing, a person, or a faith, and expectation of its realization. A classic example of the power of belief is the placebo effect. A *placebo*, pronounced pla-see'-bo, from the Latin *placeo*, meaning "to please" is a fake pill with no known effect, good or bad, unless represented to a patient or test subject as a medicine. The placebo effect is so solid scientifically that the U.S. Food and Drug Administration (FDA) requires a placebo as a control in evaluating the effectiveness of medicines.

There is a history of the origin of the placebo. As the story goes, in the early years of the 1900s there was a thriving business in patent medicines. Medical people as well as some legislators complained that almost all of them were ineffective or worse and if any of them had a feel-good effect it was due to the alcohol content. Congressional hearings were held under the leadership of a fictional Senator Placebo, who insisted that the hearings be closed to the public. But reporters managed to interview witnesses who revealed that all of the expert testimony was that patent medicines were indeed worthless. There was a hue and cry from the public for a hearings report and demands for legislative action to ban the sale of such products. After much prodding Senator Placebo made a statement. "There will be no report," he said. "I have destroyed all records of the hearings. No medical evidence was given to prove the medicines were in anyway harmful to human beings. They are safe, so why should I deny their effect?"[1]

Ever after, drugs with no effect and no harm were called placebos. After passage of the Pure Food and Drugs Act of 1906 meant to identify alcohol, opiates and other dangerous drugs, a large percentage of people continued using these "useless" remedies simply because they felt better.

An early use of placebos was in the vanished time when doctors made house calls. Whether in the doctor's office or in a home, the doctor's black bag was a handy source of remedies that would not require a sick person or a member of the family to make an arduous trip to a distant drug store to fill a prescription. The black bag always contained vials of pink or blue sugar pills for use if there was no known useful medicine for the ailment, or if the doctor determined that the best remedy would be rest and relaxation, with the comforting knowledge that something was being done by a competent doctor.

Dr. **Thomas Delbanco**, of the Harvard Medical School, says, "The placebo effect is wonderful medicine....If you make a sugar pill and charge a lot for it, it works better than a placebo for which you charge very little. And if you have certain colors on that pill, it may work even better. The placebo is one of the most powerful medicines we have. It's very hard to tell sometimes whether what we're doing is more than the placebo effect."[2, 3]

The powerful effect of the placebo is a mystery that is only partially explained by the knowledge that the brain is highly susceptible to suggestion. Says **Jon Kabat-Zinn**, founder and director of the Stress Reduction Clinic at the University of Massachusetts Medical Center, "To call what happens 'the placebo effect' is just to give a name to something we don't understand." Dr. Benson says, "...the interaction between the physician and the patient is probably the most important factor."[4]

The effect of the believable on healing was told by Mark Twain, a.k.a. Samuel Clemens (1835-1910), former Mississippi River steamboat pilot, world traveler, renowned writer, and humorist. He told how Tom Sawyer removed warts by burying a cat at midnight under the light of a full moon. Most readers of *The Adventures of Tom Sawyer* probably viewed the amusing tale as superstition or simply nonsense.[5] But in times past, skin conditions and warts in particular were favorite targets of "home remedies." While warts seem to be a poor choice to evaluate remedies, warts have long been thought to have an unexplained psychological relationship to their owners. Warts come and go, and often disappear for no apparent reason. Besides, a virus was found to be associated with warts, suggesting that it might be of interest to use warts in a scientific study of the influence of mental conditions on virus-induced diseases.

There are people who learned about the power of belief in health and healing but used the power, instead, for the vilest of evils. Voodoo, sometimes called black magic or sorcery, is thought to have originated in Africa where the powerful influence of voodoo over life and death is commonly practiced. It soon became a practice in the West Indies, especially Haiti, and is said to have been adopted in various forms by the indigenous people in parts of South America, Australia and some of the Pacific Islands.

Voodoo is quick death to the victim of a spell cast by someone who is accepted by the community as having the mysterious power. Typically, death follows within a few hours after pointing a bone at the victim or by using some other symbol or expression of doom. Voodoo has been observed and described by several well qualified scientists. One of the early observers was **Walter B. Cannon**, a Harvard University physiologist who became prominent for, among other discoveries, determining the secretion and role of adrenaline under the stimulation of fear or anger. Cannon visited the Maori aborigines of New Zealand and saw the "unmitigated terror" created when *tapu* (taboo) was imposed by tribal leaders. Dr. **Herbert Benson** in his book, *The Mind/Body Effect*, points out that the success of voodoo depends on the victim being aware of the spell and the strength of the victim's belief in voodoo magic.[6, 7, 8, 9]

Lest anyone think that ceremonial murder is confined to uneducated primitive people, Americans remember what is known as the Salem Witch Trials of the 1690s. The town of Salem is located on a harbor sixteen miles northeast of Boston. A servant of the local minister was a West Indian slave girl named **Tituba** who related tales of voodoo to a group of young girls and women. They were so terrified by the stories that they shivered and let out screams at night. They were examined by a physician who said they were bewitched. Tituba and two of the other women were accused of being witches and were sentenced to death. But that wasn't enough to satisfy the devout people of Salem. The witchcraft trials continued for about a year during which nineteen women, declared guilty as witches, were hanged on Gallows Hill and one was "pressed" to death. The presiding judge was **Samuel Sewall** (1652-1730). Five years after the trials he openly confessed that he had been wrong and considered himself more at fault than the other judges in the case. He went on to be appointed, in 1718, to chief justice of the superior court of judicature.[10]

The FDA has the responsibility to approve or disapprove all new medicines before being marketed. Participants in a trial to determine the effectiveness of a medicine are not told whether they are being given a placebo or the test medicine, although they may know that they can be given either one. The placebo and the medicine are made to look alike, and in a well organized trial, patients are selected with comparable symptoms. Half of them are given the drug and half the placebo. A good clinical trial will be *double-blind*, that is, neither the test evaluators nor the tested knows which individuals receive the placebo instead of the medicine. A third party keeps a record of who gets which and keeps the information confidential until the evaluations are completed. The placebo effect may be small or large depending on circumstances. Claims have been made that the placebo can account for as much as a fourth or a third of the medicinal effect. The new drug, itself, will be expected to have some placebo effect. If the drug and the placebo are equally effective, the conclusion would be that the drug is worthless. This poses an unresolved dilemma.[11]

Would it be logical to conclude that a placebo showing, say 20% effectiveness, should be discarded as a treatment? An obvious advantage of placebos is the absence of side effects. Doctors no longer give or prescribe placebos to patients because they think it would be unethical to fool them that way. They think that the doctor would be obligated to tell the patient that he or she is being given a placebo, in which case it would no longer be a placebo. That view may be valid. The FDA often approves several medicines to treat an ailment. Which one will be of value in a particular case is often a shot in the dark that runs the risk of causing more sickness than it cures. Should doctors tell patients that side effects (i.e., poisonous effects) may make them worse? The statement would probably have a negative placebo effect, and would detract from the patient's confidence in the physician.

Many of the writers and lecturers on the relation between mind and health are physicians. **Deepak Chopra**,M.D. a popular advocate of healthful living, demonstrated the widespread appeal of a belief in the mind's dominion over the body and the yearning for something more than blunt physical remedies such as drugs and surgery for healing and health. According to writer **Tony Perry**, in 1997, Chopra estimated his annual gross at $15 million from his 19 books translated into 25 languages, lectures, CDs, videos, seminars and related enterprises. Born in India,

Chopra was the son of a British-trained cardiologist. He studied medicine at the All India Institute of Medical Sciences, and came to the United States at the age of 23 to practice medicine. A believer in Ayurvedic healing (a traditional Hindu system of medicine practiced in India since the first century, A.D. using combinations of herbs, purgatives, rubbing oils, and so forth, in treating diseases), he brought with him the Eastern perspective that integrates with Western medical practice. A remarkably articulate and charismatic lecturer, Chopra comes across to some people as vague and unfocused. But in the face of being accused by a TV host of purveying "preposterous psychobabble," obviously many people find his teaching a pathway to spiritual fulfillment and a healthier life. In his popular book, *Perfect Health: The Complete Mind/Body Guide*, Chopra offered a somewhat metaphysical discussion of his beliefs.[12, 13]

Herbert Benson, a physician, associate professor at the Harvard Medical School, and president and founder of the Mind/Body Medical Institute, achieved wide public recognition for experiments in which he recorded the bodily calm of what he called the "relaxation response," described in his 1975 book of that name.[14] In his 1996 book, *Timeless Healing*, he further describes the relaxation response and adds the concept of "remembered wellness."[15] What Benson calls remembered wellness is akin to both the placebo effect and autosuggestion in that it draws on the natural ability of the mind and body to heal itself. Herbert Benson and **Mark D. Epstein** described three components of remembered wellness:[16] 1. Belief and expectancy on the part of the patient. 2. Belief and expectancy on the part of the caregiver. 3. Belief and expectancy generated by a relationship between the patient and the caregiver.

It's easily demonstrated that meditation calms the nerves and promotes relaxation. Different people prefer different techniques: yoga, tai chi, chanting, Zen meditation, mantras, alpha biofeedback, rural retreats, long walks, tribal dances, communal worship, prayer, and various methods of relaxation. A classic model for relaxation was given by Dr. **David Harold Fink** in his 1943 book, *Release from Nervous Tension*.[17] Dr. **Walter C. Alvarez** of the Mayo Clinic, a widely read columnist, followed in 1958 with, *Live at Peace With Your Nerves*.[18] Both Fink and Alvarez pointed out that the connection between the body and mind is not a one-way street. The body "talks back."

CHAPTER 37

FAITH HEALERS

A spectacular demonstration of faith healing is at the Roman Catholic shrine at Lourdes, located near the foothills of the Pyrenees in southwestern France. Worshipers believe that here in 1858 the **Virgin Mary** appeared to a peasant girl, **Bernadette Soubirous**, now known as **Saint Bernadette**. At the grotto where the vision occurred there is a beautiful church called the Rosary, and a statue of the Virgin. Thousands of people visit the shrine every year, leaving gifts. Some leave their crutches or other evidence of their cures. Some bathe in the sacred waters of the grotto spring, expecting a miracle to restore them to health. Although they come year-round, many French Roman Catholics make a pilgrimage to the shrine for ceremonies on August 20 of each year. The shrine at Lourdes attracts more than 2,000,000 pilgrims a year. The underground Basilica of St. Pius X, opened in 1958, is the second largest Roman Catholic church, exceeded only by St. Peter's in Rome.[1]

Mary Baker Eddy (1821-1910), founder of the Christian Science Church, forged an exceptionally strong link between mind control and religious faith. Her book, *Science and Health with Key to the Scriptures*, was offered as giving the complete meaning of Christianity. According to **George Channing**, who was a Christian Science lecturer, teacher, and practitioner, "God is divine Mind…and Mind is all that exists….Spirit is eternal and real; matter is an unreal illusion subject to decay and dissolution." Christian scientists believe strongly in the power of prayer. Faith and expectation of a positive outcome are evident in Christian Science belief. Says Channing, "Christian Science holds that good is infinite, that sin, death, and disease are unreal, and that evil is a delusion."[3]

Mary Baker Patterson Glover Eddy was born and grew up on a farm near Concord, New Hampshire. She married in 1843 at the age of 22 to **George Washington Glover** who died before the birth of her only child. She remained a widow for ten years during which, it is said, she had periods of nervous disorder illnesses. In 1853 she married **Daniel Patterson**, an itinerant dentist. He deserted her and her child, after which she eventually obtained a divorce. Meanwhile she became interested in the teaching of **Phineas Parkhurst Quimby**, a clockmaker who experimented with mesmerism. He then practiced a form of faith healing that he called Christian Science, "the science of health and happiness."

In 1875 Mary published her chief writing, *Science and Health with Key to the Scriptures*. In 1877 she married **Asa G. Eddy** who helped her establish the Church of Christ Scientist. In 1908 she founded a daily newspaper, *The Christian Science Monitor*.[4, 5] Christian Science attracted many followers. It was controversial because in illness the faithful were asked to rely only on faith and to reject medical help.

One of the most influential proponents of mind over matter, positive thinking, and faith was **Ernest Holmes**, founder of the Church of Religious Science. In his book, *The Science of Mind*, he says, "Man, by thinking, can bring into his experience whatever he desires….all thought is creative, according to the nature, impulse, emotion, or conviction behind the thought."[6] Holmes advocated meditation and prayer, and the power of words. He emphasized faith and expectation.[7, 8]

Norman Vincent Peale, minister of Marble Collegiate Church in New York City. Peale was a dynamic speaker who lectured extensively to business groups as well as at spiritual meetings. Peale's book, *The Power of Positive Thinking*, and other writings and lectures, linked positive thinking to faith in God and the teachings of Jesus.[9, 10] His book, proclaimed "The great inspirational best-seller of our time," was offered as "a practical guide to mastering the problems of everyday living." Coué's recommendation (discussed in chapter 38) received worldwide attention, but it was not taken seriously by everyone. The idea in modified form was revived half a century later by others, most prominently by Peale.

An early proponent of the power of faith was the New York cleric **Emmet Fox**, who conducted Sunday morning services at the Biltmore and Astor Hotels, the old Hippodrome, the Manhattan Opera House, and Carnegie Hall. Among his more persuasive writings was a 6-page booklet entitled *The Golden Key* and a later book, *Stake Your Claim*[11, 12] in which he ascribed to God "The Divine Law" that would answer prayer. He advised readers to stop dwelling on problems and, instead, to defer to a higher power. He told them to pay no attention to what things at first may appear to be, and advised against negative thinking. He recommended giving thanks and to try to feel thankful, then to forget about it until next day.

Belief and expectancy, we've already seen, are components of positive suggestibility. **Herbert Benson** contends that the healing effects of what he calls "remembered wellness" are helped by a belief in God.[13] Do religious people live longer and healthier lives, on average, than non-believers? Mormons and Seventh Day Adventists are among the healthier groups, maybe only partly due to their healthful life styles.

Belief in prayer can contribute powerfully to suggestibility. Faith in prayer is a major part of most religions, although it is practiced in different ways. The idea that the combination of prayer and belief has invincible power was put forth nearly two thousand years ago by **Jesus of Nazareth** who was quoted as saying, "Have faith in God....Therefor whatever things you desire when you pray, believe that you receive them and you shall have them."[14] It was written two or three hundred years earlier in the Book of Proverbs, the book of wise sayings, "Trust in the Lord with all your heart; and lean not on your own understanding."[15]

Almost all inspirational advocates of prayer and positive thinking mention the importance of imagination, or as **Norman Vincent Peale** puts it, "the expectation of miracles." A writer and lecturer named **Neville** was another exponent of imagination. In his book, *Awakened Imagination*, he says "Imagination is the very gateway to reality."[16]

An aspect that is not usually mentioned by advocates of positive thinking is that suggestions have the power to give good or bad results. We are bombarded daily with positive and negative suggestions. Some things we yearn for may not be good for us or for others. There's a wise saying, "Be careful what you pray for—you might get it."

Participation in group activities bring the benefits of fellowship, companionship, and other social needs to a naturally gregarious animal. Many believe that faith in the power of God reinforces what an associate professor at Harvard Medical School, **Herbert Benson**, calls "remembered wellness," which to be effective has to be backed up by *belief and expectations*.[17] **Dr. David Smith**, a physician, saw religion as an aid to healing. Formerly senior vice president to Parkland Memorial Hospital in Dallas, Texas, and CEO and medical director of the Community Oriented Primary Care (COPC) of the hospital, Dr. Smith said of religion, "It's a very powerful force in the community....we often turn to the church, which becomes part of the therapeutic process."[18]

Belief is essential for faith healing, and for self healing. Norman Cousins in his book, *Anatomy of an Illness*, tells how an experience as a youngster set his mind on a trend that later in life enabled him to cure himself of a supposedly "incurable" disease. At the age of ten he was sent to a tuberculosis sanitarium. He was frail and underweight, and it seemed logical to believe that he was afflicted with a terrible disease. It developed that the doctor had mistakenly interpreted the X-ray picture showing normal calcification as the presence of TB. At that time X-ray technology had not become reliable. Norman spent six months at the sanitarium during which the patients divided into two groups, those who were confident that they could overcome their problem and those who resigned themselves to a long, possibly fatal illness. Those who were optimistic avoided the other group, and tried to recruit newcomers before the pessimists could influence them. The outcome was that a much higher percentage of the boys in Norman's group were discharged as cured. The experience made Norman aware of the power of the mind and faith in his ability to overcome disease.[19]

The power of belief is seen in Voodoo. **Dr. Walter B. Cannon** tells of a letter he received from Dr. **S.M. Lambert**, a fellow physician who was visiting a mission at Mona Mona in North Queensland. Many of the natives there had been converted but there was a group of non-converts on the fringe that included **Nebo**, a witch doctor. **Rob**, the chief helper at the mission, was ailing and the missionary asked Dr. Lambert to examine him. After a thorough examination the doctor said that he could find no fever, no pain, and no symptoms of disease although Rob was obviously seriously ill and very weak. The missionary said that Nebo had pointed a bone at Rob who was convinced it meant he must die. Dr. Lambert and the missionary went to Nebo and told him that if anything were to happen to Rob, Nebo's food supply would be cut off and he and his group would be driven off the mission. Nebo promptly went to see Rob to tell him that it was all a mistake, that he did not actually point a bone at him, and it was just all in fun. Dr. Lambert reported that Rob's recovery was almost instantaneous.

Rob went back to work that evening, happy and back to full physical strength.

Dr. Lambert reported that in a similar case the victim of a voodoo spell was less fortunate. **Dr. P.S. Clarke** was treating Kanakas, natives employed on a sugar plantation in North Queensland. One of the Kanakas came to Dr. Clarke's hospital and complained that he would die in a few days. A thorough examination gave no indication of disease, so Dr. Clarke brought in the foreman of the plantation crew, thinking he might give the suffering man some hope of recovery. When the foreman came to the man's bedside he looked at the patient, turned to Dr. Clarke and said "Yes, doctor, close up him die." (He is near death). The man died the next morning.[20, 21]

In historic days people thought of a god or gods as having a special interest in their lives especially in times of danger or stress. Roman soldiers had Mars, the war god. Similarly today, people in various segments of society rely on faith in God for comfort, protection or success. The World War II saying, "There are no atheists in foxholes" went unchallenged. In sports, a boxer may cross himself before a fight in the presumed knowledge that God knows something about slipping punches or landing a cross right. **Tommy Lasorda**, former manager of the Los Angeles Dodgers, always attentive to team morale, would talk of "the Big Dodger in the sky", presumably in full uniform trimmed in Dodger blue. It can be taken as a subtle reminder of the universal hope for support beyond ones own limited capabilities. Sports writer **Jim Murray** said, "God is a golfer, every weekend hacker is sure, probably a five handicap but maybe scratch." Murray fantasized God challenging the immortal **Ben Hogan** to a match.[22]

Coaches, managers, trainers, and owners use methods that each thinks will have the strongest motivation. Argentina's **Diego Maradona** takes his soccer team to a catholic mass before a big game. The American **Landon Donovan** makes the sign of the cross before a penalty kick, and Mexico's **Javier Hernandez** kneels with his arms outstretched in prayer before the start of a match. Soccer teams' need for help came into prominence during the 2010 World Cup competition when the Confederation of African Football banned *traditional healers* from associating with the teams. One of them was **Kenneth Nephawe**, known as a *sangoma*, a practitioner of herbal medicine, divination and counseling. He is also called a *juju man*, though he prefers to be known as a "traditional healer." The West African nation soccer team, the best in Africa, claimed that the injury keeping midfielder

Michael Essien out of action was the result of a spell cast by his father in revenge for being neglected. The Rev. **Osei Kofi**, a former national league team star, said a Ghana club team had spent more than $60,000 last season on what he called "superstitions." A journalist said that at Soccer City, the main World Cup venue, 300 sangomas gathered to sacrifice an ox in a traditional good-luck ceremony. The move to ban the traditional healers was made during preparation for the World Cup which would be the first to be played in Africa. They had in mind that sangomas are viewed in other parts of the world as witch doctors, which to many Africans is ignorance and in a way arrogance because in many areas of the continent traditional healing is part of the fabric of society and a vital part of the fight against diseases including AIDS. According to the South African Tourist Bureau eight in 10 South Africans visit a traditional healer at least three times a year.[23]

Faith healers are common in the historical landscape. According to scripture a famous healer in biblical times was **Jesus of Nazareth**, whose miracle cures along with his words of wisdom attracted a huge following.

And his fame went all through Syria. (Matthew 4:24)
And there followed him great multitudes of people. (Matthew 4:25)

Jesus thought it was prudent to avoid publicity. After curing a leper:

….Jesus saith unto him, See thou tell no man; but go thy way, shew thyself to the priest, and offer the gift that Moses commanded. (Matthew 8:4)

Jesus crossed over to the east side of the Sea of Galilee.

And when he was come to the other side…there met him two possessed with devils…. (Matthew 8:28)

There followed a description of Jesus casting out the devils, who at their own request changed into a herd of swine that plunged into the Sea of Galilee and drowned.[2] After Jesus' Sermon on the Mount:

…there came unto him a centurion (an officer in charge of 100 soldiers), *beseeching him,* (Matthew 8:5)

And saying, Lord, my servant lieth at home sick of the palsy. (Matthew 8:6)

The centurion begged Jesus not to bother coming personally, but to say the healing word from a distance. Jesus did so, saying,

...I have not found so great faith, no, not in Israel. (Matthew 8:10)

There is the story of Jesus raising the dead son of a widow:

And he said, young man, I say unto thee, Arise. (Luke 7:14)
And he that was dead sat up, and began to speak... (Luke 7:15)

But the crowning achievement of Jesus' ministry was a call for him to go to Judea where a friend was seriously ill as told by John:

Now a certain man was sick, named Lazarus, of Bethany, the town of Mary and her sister Martha. (John 11:1)
Therefore his sisters sent unto him, saying, Lord, behold, he whom thou lovest is sick. (John 11:3)

But when Jesus arrived, Lazurus was dead and buried and had been in the tomb for four days. Jesus had the stone blocking the tomb rolled away.

And... he (Jesus) cried with a loud voice, Lazarus, come forth. (John 11:43)
And he that was dead came forth.... (John 11:44)

Evangelism became popular in the United States during the early part of the twentieth century. Evangelists, some of the faith healers, often without a particular denominational affiliation, would sometimes conduct services in a miniature circus tent setup on a vacant lot. The more successful ones would form an alliance with a church or join a denomination. An early popular evangelist was **Billy Sunday** (William Ashley Sunday, 1862-1935), born in Ames, Iowa. His original career was in professional baseball from 1883 to 1891 with the Chicago White Stockings, Pittsburgh Alleghenys, and the Philadelphia Phillies. It was during his baseball days that he was converted and went to work for the YMCA. He became a Presbyterian minister in 1903. He traveled widely as an evangelist and drew large crowds wherever he appeared throughout the country.[24]

The most popular evangelist, well liked and respected worldwide, is **Billy Graham** (William Franklin Graham, (1918-). He graduated from Wheaton (IL) College and was ordained a minister in 1940. His early work in the United States and England for the "Youth for Christ Crusade" inspired him and his colleagues to conduct a large scale evangelistic campaign in Los Angeles in 1949. The success of the campaign convinced Graham that he should engage in a career devoted solely to large scale evangelism. He conducted campaigns in the United States, England, Scotland, and other countries in Europe, the Middle East, the Far East, and Africa. He started a radio program, "The Hour of Decision," in 1950. He appeared on television and made several films. He wrote *Peace With God* (1954), *Secret of Happiness* (1955), and *My Answer* (1960).[25]

CHAPTER 38

MESMERISM

Mesmerism, a powerful form of suggestion better known as hypnotism, was discovered or possibly rediscovered, by a German physician, **Franz Anton Mesmer** (1734-1815), who vigorously promoted the technique as a curative for various ailments although he had virtually no understanding of what was happening. Hypnotism (hypnosis) may have been a feature of ancient healing. There are cave paintings of what some anthropologists interpret as "magicians." And **Hippocrates** is said to have descended from a family of magicians[1] headed by **Asclepius**, a shadowy figure credited with being the inspiration for a cult of priests and temples. Asclepius became the Greek god of healing.

Mesmer was born in Iznang am Bodensee, Baden, Germany, on the shore of Lake Constance. He started out studying law but switched to medicine and obtained his medical degree at the University of Vienna in 1766. His interests were inclined toward whatever little-understood phenomena were attracting the interests of scientists. He thought there must be a way to use the new developments in electricity and magnetism to cure diseases. He believed that a cosmic force permeated all things including people and it could be used to influence the body and psyche of another, as physician to patient.

Mesmer believed that the force permeating people was comparable to that of a magnet. He started out by passing magnets over the bodies of his patients, many of whom were cured. He then found that he did not need the magnets, but could get the same results by passing his hands over the patient's bodies. He also used iron rods and wands. He attributed the effect to "animal magnetism," and he reasoned that sickness is caused by an interruption in the flow of animal magnetism in the body.

But Mesmer's practice in Vienna ran into trouble. His cures, widely acclaimed by himself and patients, brought notoriety, but there were also failures, and not surprisingly, complaints followed by charges of malpractice. The Vienna police, no doubt urged on by conventional medical practitioners, ordered Mesmer to move on. He went to Paris in 1778 where he founded a hospital that became immensely popular among a fashionable clientele. Mesmer found that he could induce what he called sleep in a person during which various things could happen including, he claimed, communication with the dead or other spirits. This psychic condition was called the "great sleep," induced by what eventually came to be known as *mesmerism*.

Mesmer fared no better with authorities in Paris than he did in Vienna. Orthodox doctors were enraged, and protested so vehemently that **Louis XVI** (reigned 1774-1792) appointed a commission of experts to investigate. They reported that they could find no evidence of animal magnetism. Members of the commission included **Antoine Lavoisier** (1743-1795), a prominent and respected chemist, **Joseph Guillotin** (1738-1814), inventor of the dreaded guillotine, and **Benjamin Franklin** (1706-1790), who was in Paris representing the young United States. Although Franklin concurred with the commission's appraisal, he discussed psychosomatic illnesses with remarkably modern understanding. Mesmer was forced to leave Paris in 1785. He moved to Versailles, then to Switzerland, and finally retired to the region of his native Lake Constance where he died in obscurity at the age of 81.[2]

It's clear that Mesmer was improving the health and sense of well-being of his patients by using the power of suggestion. The method was revived in a more respectable form a half century later by a Scottish surgeon, **James Braid** (1795-1860). Born at Rylawhouse, Fifeshire, Braid attended medical school at Edinburgh, but moved to Manchester, England to practice surgery. When he attended some exhibitions of mesmerism, they left him skeptical of the entire idea. But when he conducted some experiments on his own, he began to think that it had some validity. He found that a person could be put into a trance-like, apparently semiconscious, state in which he or she was exceptionally open to suggestion.[3]

Braid concluded that the phenomenon had nothing to do with animal magnetism. Instead, he said, it was a suspension of consciousness forced by the weariness of repetitive stimuli. He called it "hypnotism" from the Greek word *hypnos*, meaning "sleep." Braid's enthusiasm for a phenomenon scorned by establishment doctors damaged his reputation, but some prominent physicians became convinced of its value. A French neurologist, **Jean-Martin Charcot** (1825-1893), who studied patients with various nervous system afflictions, became especially interested in patients who showed the symptoms of a neurological problem but who had no evidence of organic disorders. Most physicians of the time dismissed such cases as "hysterical illness" or simply malingering. The term "hysterical" came from the Greek word *hystera*, for uterus, under the belief that it was mostly women who claimed to have such ailments. Charcot believed that the patients were truly suffering and undertook to treat them with hypnosis. **Sigmund Freud** (1856-1939) was intrigued with Charcot's approach and is thought by some to have influenced Freud's own search for explanations of neurotic behavior. Those who worked with hypnosis demonstrated early in the game that it could be used to make a person less aware, or even unaware, of pain. The knowledge was available for adoption of the technique by the medical profession as a standard treatment for pain. But unfortunately, or fortunately depending on one's viewpoint, the introduction of new, safe, and affective anesthetics was a dramatic breakthrough in surgery as well as for ordinary treatment of pain. Some psychologists and clinical psychologists continue to use hypnosis, but the public's interest is mainly in hypnosis as theatrical stunts.

Las Vegas entertainers caught on to the idea of making hypnotism a feature of their shows. They can be visited at several casinos on the Strip such as the Tropicana, Planet Hollywood, and Paris Las Vegas. Most of the entertainers who conduct hypnotism shows on the Strip started as comedians but took instructions in hypnosis from teachers who were skilled in the art. To hone their performance some of them became certified clinical hypnotists. Cruise ships are another venue for their shows.

Because hypnosis is probably the purest and most readily demonstrated form of suggestion, an analytical examination of it may open a window into understanding other levels of suggestion that are part of everyday life. *Webster's New World Dictionary* defines hypnosis as "A trance-like condition usually induced by another person, in which the subject is in a state of altered consciousness and responds, with certain limitations, to the suggestions of the hypnotist." This leaves some unanswered questions. What is a trance? The same dictionary defines a trance as "a state of altered consciousness, somewhat resembling sleep, during which voluntary movement is lost, as in hypnosis." But hypnosis is not sleep. Physiological measurements taken during hypnosis are nearly the same as those taken during wakefulness. Reflexes are the same as when awake, while during sleep, reflexes such as knee jerk are absent or reduced. In sleep, consciousness of the outside world is greatly diminished, whereas in hypnosis responses to outside stimuli are retained. Brain waves also resemble those during wakefulness.[4] "In the final analysis, hypnosis appears to be a condition which is neither the normal working state nor any one of the sleep stages," say psychiatrists **Barbara DeBetz** and **Gerard Sunnen**.[5] In fact, one does not have to be in a trance at all to respond to suggestions as attested by the universal belief in the power of commercial advertising. Says **Barbara Brown**, UCLA psychologist, in *New Mind, New Body*, "People with a fair amount of alpha in the EEG (please see Chapter 39) were found in those who were most susceptible to hypnosis," and "…successful learning to control alpha was accompanied by an increased susceptibility to hypnosis."

Says Brown on the medical use of hypnosis:

Both hypnosis and biofeedback (please see Chapter 39) *are capable of controlling body functions without drugs and without surgery. Now there are two fingers pointing toward the dominion of mind over matter….It is as if medicine fears the potential power of the mind….Yet if hypnosis can control bleeding as well as pain, it is a major oversight that hypnosis has not been explored scientifically and systematically for its effect on other body functions.*[6]

SELF HYPNOSIS (AUTOSUGGESTION)

The idea of giving oneself suggestions in the "waking state," that is, *autosuggestion*, was introduced and publicized early in the 20th century by **Émile Coué**. Born in 1857 in Troyes, France, Coué studied pharmacy in Paris, and returned to Troyes where he opened a drugstore. While on a visit to his wife's parents home in Nancy in 1901, he attended a lecture on hypnosis at the Nancy School of Hypnotism under **Dr. Liebault**, a leading proponent of the technique for treating patients. Coué studied diligently under Liebault and began to hold hypnotic clinics right in his drugstore. Probably most of his clients were drugstore customers, and Coué noticed that many of them improved beyond what would be expected from their medicines alone. He also noticed that only about 10% of his subjects went into a complete hypnotic state. This led him to believe that the patients gave themselves the suggestions while fully awake, and he eventually concluded that hypnotism was not necessary at all. In other words, the subjects could obtain the beneficial results themselves by conscious *autosuggestion*.[8, 9, 10]

Coué and his wife moved to Nancy in 1910 and opened their home, free of charge, to anyone who needed help. In his books, *Self Mastery Through Conscious Autosuggestion*, published in 1922, and *My Method*, published in 1923, Coué advocated repeating the phrase, "Every day and in every way, I am becoming better and better." He recommended repeating this every night twenty or thirty times or more before dropping off to sleep in a low voice just loud enough to be heard by oneself. It is not necessary, Coué said, to refer to specific problems or details. "Let the subconscious take over," he said.

In view of differences in the way psychologists describe hypnosis, we can do no better than to take the word of psychologist **Clark L. Hull** who maintained that the only difference between the hypnotized and non hypnotized state was that people under hypnosis are more suggestible, that is, they are in a state of hypersuggestibility.[7] **Hull**, writing in 1933, then an experimental psychologist at Yale University, discussed the distinction between self hypnosis and suggestion. "The difference," he observed, "between the hypnotic state and the normal is a quantitative rather than a qualitative one. Despite the widespread and long-standing belief to the contrary, the author is convinced that no phenomenon whatever can be produced by hypnosis that cannot be produced to lesser degrees by suggestions given in the normal waking condition."[11]

Frank S. Caprio, a psychiatrist, and **Joseph R. Berger**, a psychologist, point out that hypnotic suggestions can come from within. In their book, *Helping yourself to self-hypnosis*, they define hypnosis as "a state of heightened suggestibility," and they tell how to use it to advantage. The first step they call for is what they call "auto-relaxation," followed by "auto-suggestion" in which there is voluntary acceptance of a suggestion. They say, "Just as we are susceptible to being influenced by others we are also susceptible to being influenced by our own thoughts."[12]

In today's medical therapy with hypnosis, the emphasis is on *training* people to use *auto-suggestion*. **Dr. Andrew Weil**, clinical professor of medicine and director of the Program on Integrative Medicine at the University of Arizona, is a leader in teaching and practicing a combination of traditional and non-traditional methods of healthful living and healing.[13] Dr. Weil and a colleague, **Dr. Steven Gurgevich**, a PhD psychologist on the faculty of the University of Arizona's College of Medicine, offer a two volume CD, entitled *Heal Yourself with Medical Hypnosis*. They say there is "proof positive that it can help ease chronic pain, lessen the side effects of chemotherapy, counteract anxiety and sleep disorders, and much more."

Remarkable results were obtained by **Dr. Karen Olness**, who was Professor of Pediatrics, Family Medicine, and International Health at Case Western Reserve University. She taught biofeedback and self-hypnosis to children. She found that children with migraine headaches can learn how to use their imaginations to reduce the frequency and severity of migraines. The technique is for them to regularly practice a relaxation imagery exercise. Olness asked the children to think about something they are interested in and like and enjoy. She lets them decide what to imagine. One 10-year old girl imagined that she was playing tennis. Says Olness, "I teach self-hypnosis to the children, but I think that needs some definition. In the course of their day-to-day play, children probably go in and out of a hypnotic state....Many athletic teams have a format identical to ours, but call it a biofeedback exercise or a relaxation exercise. A relaxation exercise may induce a temporary alteration of awareness." Olness says that biofeedback takes a lot of practice to be successful: "It took me two months of daily practice to develop what I would call excellent skills in pain control. Children learn much more quickly." Olness had surgery—a 45 minute procedure—and used self-regulation of pain as her only anesthesia. What was going on in her mind? "I was focused and concentrated," she says, "....I was thinking about a favorite memory...being on the farm where I grew up."[14]

Self hypnosis is less easily achieved than conventional hypnosis simply because it requires discipline and practice. However, most psychologists agree that all hypnosis is essentially self hypnosis, in which a state of altered consciousness is induced by either a practitioner or oneself.[15]

CHAPTER 39

BIOFEEDBACK

The body is a dynamo of electrical activity, producing enough energy to transmit information by way of the nervous system from one part of the organism to another with the split-second velocity of an electro-chemical wave. Messages are propagated along the nerve fibers by what is called the *sodium-potassium pump*. In the resting stage it keeps sodium (Na+) high along the outer edge of the nerve fiber, and potassium (K+) high along the inside. When a signal arrives for a message (like, say, stubbing a toe or stepping on a tack) the concentrations of Na+ and K+ switch sides rapidly, moving in a wave that sweeps along the nerve fiber with a velocity of up to 120 m/sec (meters per second) depending on the location of the nerve.[1, 2, 3]

Most of the electrical activity is beyond conscious control, such as blood pressure, heart rate, relaxation, nervous tension, anxiety, or fear, or other emotions. But hooking ourselves up to instruments can make us aware of what's happening and, with practice through biofeedback, enable us to control much of what may be troubling.[4]

The highest concentration of the body's electrical activity is in the brain, which produces prodigious amounts of electrical discharges that can be measured as brain waves by attaching an electroencephalograph (EEG) to the scalp. When the pioneer brain wave researcher **Hans Berger** noticed a surge of brain wave activity it seemed natural for him to call these first brain waves observed *alpha waves*. The alpha waves disappeared when the subjects opened their eyes. (Most wave researchers test their subjects with their eyes closed). The waves reappear in large swells when they close their eyes. The alpha waves also disappeared when the subjects engaged in mental activity requiring concentration and effort.[5] The duration of an alpha wave is roughly 100 milliseconds, that is, a frequency of one every 0.1 second or 10 waves per second. Of course, brain waves represent a continuous rhythmic change in electrical activity. The energy of alpha waves ranges from 20 to 150 microvolts, that is, 20 to 150 millionths of a volt.[6] This compares to house current of about 115 volts. There is a connection between large amounts of alpha waves and meditation. Early reports showed that practicing students of Zen and yoga developed large amounts of alpha waves immediately after beginning meditation, but that brain electrical activity gradually changed to the slower *theta waves*, typically associated with such diverse forms of behavior as drowsiness, dreaming, and assimilation of new information. Some advocates called alpha activity instant Zen.[7] Researchers saw the possibility of using brain waves in biofeedback to control body functions when a pioneering Frenchwoman, **Thérèse Brosse**, took a portable electrocardiogram (ECG) machine to India in 1935 and returned with graphic evidence that a veteran meditator could influence cardiac rhythm to the extent of stopping the heart completely for a few seconds.

The electrical activity in muscle is also useful in biofeedback. An electromyograph (EMG) can be used for learning relaxation and anxiety control. Determinations of body functions other than electrical activity have been extensively studied in biofeedback, primarily temperature, heart rate, and blood pressure. Self monitoring using biofeedback has been applied to a wide variety of conditions, including hypertension, anxiety, tension headaches, migraine, cardiac arrhythmia, asthma, epilepsy, and many others.

Barbara Brown, pharmacologist and neurophysiologist, was a pioneer in experimenting and developing biofeedback and methods of learning to control body functions by monitoring one's own brain waves. Brown discovered that the brain emits at least four kinds of waves that depend on the brain's activity at the time of measurement: *delta*, the sleep pattern; *theta*, linked to creative activity pattern; *beta*, the mental concentration pattern; and *alpha*, relating to a relaxed state. Brown thought that if people could relate physical sensations to each wave type, they could learn to produce the various states at will.

Brown graduated from Ohio State University in 1938, and obtained a Ph.D. in Pharmacology from the University of Cincinnati in 1950. She became head of the division of pharmacology at William S. Merrell Company, then worked for Riker Labs, Inc., as a research pharmacologist while consulting on neurophysiology at the Veterans Administration hospital in Sepulveda, California (now North Hills). She then became an associate professor of pharmacology at UC Irvine, California, chief experimental physiologist at the VA hospital, lecturer at the department of psychiatry, UCLA Medical School, and pharmacologist at the Center for Health Science, UCLA.

One of the most easily monitored organs of the body is the skin. Barbara Brown, in her book *New Mind, New Body*, writes about "skin talk." She says the skin is not talking about the skin, it's talking about the mind: "And what we can learn in skin biofeedback is not control of the skin, but control of emotions and mental activity." It would be just as correct to call monitoring the skin "sweat talk" because most of the variation in electrical signals from the skin are from the sweat glands. The sweat glands broadcast emotions: fear, anxiety, worry, tension, relaxation, passion, excitement, happiness, tranquility, and their degrees of intensity. Even when there is no visible sweat, the electrical signals are present because there is constant chemical communication between the inside and outside through the sweat glands. The flow of the electrolytes, sodium and potassium, are important in the communication network throughout the body as well as in the skin. The electrical signal can be measured as either voltage or current.

Skin talk will tell if a person is lying. It was used in lie detectors even before the discovery of biofeedback. It's clear that the skin's electrical activity originates in the brain and signals the emotions of the moment. A person wired to a device to listen to skin talk, known as the galvanic skin response (GSR), can learn something about the mental or physical state that's apt to produce a desired result such as relaxation. A curious finding is that skin talk is louder and clearer on the right side of the body than on the left side, irrespective of whether one is right- or left-handed. This may or may not be related to the fact that the speech center is on the left side of the brain, which controls many of the functions of the right side of the body.[8]

Biofeedback, although one of the best ways to demonstrate the power of the mind over physiology, has never achieved its potential usefulness, probably because learning it requires the subject to be hooked up to instruments. The body contains many feedback systems that self-regulate physiological functions: temperature, pupil adjustment for light, and muscle movement for near and far vision, perspiration, sneezing, heart rate accommodation to relaxation or exertion, breathing rate and depth, blood pressure, secretion of saliva, relaxation of sphincter for urinating, scratching an itch, constriction and relaxation of thousands of muscle fibers for an infinite number of tasks, secretion of hormones when needed and shutdown when there is enough, and more.

It has long been the practice in medicine to measure conditions that are useful in diagnosis and treatment: temperature, blood pressure, heart rate, blood cell counts, and more recently, complicated chemical profiles of the blood. Biofeedback procedure enables the subject to become aware of the internal self. It consists of continuously monitoring a feature of the body's activity, usually by a flickering light, variable tone, a scratching pen, or electrical conductivity of the skin in a way that makes it possible to sense desirable and undesirable states. If the subject is alerted to his or her mental or physical attitude or thoughts at the moment the light flashes or the bell sounds—such as being calm or relaxed—the subject can consciously give oneself the suggestion to return to that attitude or thought that produced the calmness or relaxation. In this way, a person can *learn* to control internal functions.

Bio-feedback Training (BFT) differs from most of the techniques in that it depends on instruments to measure the body's response to thoughts and emotions. Thus informed, the mind learns how to cope with them, for example, tension headache treatment with auto-suggestion. Barbara Brown, a leader in developing bio-feedback, describes it, "Bio-feedback is interacting with the interior self."

Autogenic training (AG), a technique for profound muscle relaxation involving a form of psychotherapy using hypnosis was developed in the 1920s by **Oskar Vogt**, a German psychiatrist who found that patients were able to induce a hypnotic state by autosuggestion. He determined that, with the help of clues from patients, a little time spent every day on "auto-hypnotic" exercises relieved fatigue and tension. Another psychiatrist, **J. H. Schultz**, expanded and revised Vogt's method in a procedure that required several months of practice after which the patient was switched to meditation exercises. Schultz was highly successful, and AG was popular in Europe, but it never caught on in the United States probably because of "the very long time involved in treatment."[9]

Medical hypnosis is demonstrated to be effective as an anesthetic but it is mostly ignored by the medical profession, so serious studies of its effectiveness are in short supply. Time, practice, and training can hardly compete with the convenience of pills and injections, although there are circumstances in which auto-suggestion would be better for the patient. "No one knows how far the control can go," says Barbara Brown. "Both hypnosis and bio-feedback are capable of controlling body functioning without drugs and without surgery. Now there are two fingers pointing to the dominion of mind over matter, and a third, acupuncture, has emerged from its eastern medicine chest."[10]

CHAPTER 40

A SELF HEALER

A famous case of self-healing was described by **Norman Cousins** in his book *Anatomy of an Illness*[1] with an elaboration of his philosophy and opinions in a subsequent book, *The Celebration of Life*.[2] Cousins became editor of *Saturday Review* in 1940, a position he held for more than 30 years, then became its editorial chairman.

In July, 1964, Cousins went to the Soviet Union as chairman of an American delegation to consider problems of cultural exchange. The conferences had been held in Leningrad after which they went to Moscow for more meetings. Their hotel was in a residential area. Cousins' room was on the second floor. Each night, diesel trucks plied back and forth to a housing project in round the clock construction. Because it was summer the windows were wide open. Cousins slept uneasily each night and felt somewhat nauseated in arising. Cousins' wife who was with him on the trip had no ill effects.

The meetings had not been casual. Paperwork had kept Cousins up late nights. The last night in Moscow had been an experience of almost total frustration. A reception had been arranged by the chairman of the Soviet delegation at his dacha (country cottage) located thirty or forty miles outside the city. They had asked Cousins to arrive an hour early to tell the Soviet Delegates about the individual Americans who were coming for the dinner. Cousins was told that a driver from the government automobile pool would pick him up at the hotel at 3:30 pm which would give ample time for Cousins to arrive at the dacha by 5:00.

However, at 6:00 Cousins found that he was in open country on the wrong side of Moscow, eighty miles off course. The driver was unhurried. They didn't arrive at the dacha until 9:00 P.M. The host's wife was desolate.

She had warmed up the soup several times. The flight back to the States the next day was tiring. He had a slight fever and the plane was crowded, and by the time they cleared New York and headed back to Connecticut there was an uneasiness deep in Cousins' bones. A week later he was hospitalized. As Cousins looked back on his trouble he concluded that he had suffered adrenal exhaustion. Cousins remembered having read Walter B. Cannon's book, *Wisdom of the Body*, that he called "homeostasis," and Hans Selye's book, *The Stress of Life* in which he pointed out that adrenal exhaustion could be caused by emotional tension or suppressed rage. Cousins pondered both the negative effects and probable positive effects of the two opposing states of mind, and concluded that it would be helpful to discuss his ideas with his physician, **Dr. William Hitzig**. A general feeling of "achiness" deepened and within a week it was hard for him to move his neck, arms, hands, fingers and legs. His sedimentation rate (the speed with which red blood cells settle in a test tube, measured in millimeters per hour), was over 80. In routine illness the "sed" rate might be 30 or 40. If it goes over 60 or 70, the physician knows that he is not dealing with an ordinary health problem. When Cousin's sed rate reached 88 he was hospitalized, and within a week it was up to 115, a level generally taken to mean a critical condition.

Dr. **William Hitzig**, long time friend of Cousins, called in various specialists as consultants. He told Cousins that there was no agreement on a precise diagnosis but there was a consensus that he was suffering from a serious collagen illness. Collagen is the fibrous substance that binds cells together, also called connective tissue. There are many diseases in which collagen disorders play a part, for example, some types of arthritic and rheumatic diseases. Experts at Dr. **Howard Rusk**'s rehabilitation clinic in New York gave Cousins' illness a name: *ankylosing spondylitis*. Dr. Hitzig told Cousins that a specialist had given him one chance in five hundred of a full recovery.

Said Cousins, "In a sense, then, I was coming unstuck." He had difficulty moving his limbs, or turning over in bed. Nodules appeared on his body, gravel-like material under the skin. At the low point of his illness his jaws were almost locked. Cousins did some deep thinking and made a decision. "If I'm going to be that one in five hundred," he thought, "I'll have to take some action." He recalled that his business in Moscow on his trip had been extremely stressful and exhausting. He speculated that it had drained his adrenal gland, and cited **Hans Selye**'s book, *The Stress of Life*,³ in which he said that adrenal exhaustion could be caused by emotional tension such as frustration or suppressed rage. Cousins became annoyed at the hospital's operation and the number and frequency of tests. For example, four technicians from four different departments came on the same day and each took large samples of blood, quantities that would threaten the welfare of a healthy person. When all four came the next day Cousins turned them away. He had a sign posted on his door saying that he would give only one specimen every three days and that he expected the different departments to draw from that sample. He made note of all the shortcomings of his hospital stay, and soon became convinced that "a hospital is no place for a person who is seriously ill." Dr. Hitzig readily agreed to have him transferred to a nearby hotel where he wouldn't be persuaded to take the huge doses of medicines they had been feeding him, for example 26 aspirin tablets and 12 phenylbutazone tablets a day, as well as massive doses of sleeping pills and other medications. Cousins wisely questioned the effects of being saturated with so many toxic chemicals. While still in the hospital, a friend had a projector installed so he could watch movies of his choice. At the hotel he could watch them any time of the night or day without disturbing other patients. His favorites were comedy movies that could make him laugh, such as old Marx Brothers films, and the spoofing TV movies, "Candid Camera." He found that ten minutes of belly laughter had an anesthetic effect that gave him at least two hours of pain free sleep. When that wore off he would repeat with another funny movie. In short, laughter was good medicine.

A second thing that proved to be crucial in his recovery was ascorbic acid. When Cousins asked about massive doses of vitamin C, Dr. Hitzig said he knew of cases in the hospital in which patients had been given up to 3 grams of the vitamin by intramuscular injection but warned him that large doses could cause kidney damage or even damage to some of the blood vessels. Cousins wanted 25 grams! But how to do it in a way the body could handle it? He thought of delivering it to the blood stream by slow drip over three or four hours, a common procedure for medications and nutrients. They started with 10 grams of ascorbic acid and increased it gradually over several days to 25 grams. The sedimentation rate dropped dramatically. (Cousins didn't say, but one would presume that ascorbic acid was already being given to him in what would be deemed a safe dose, probably no more than one gram per day, because it's well known that the vitamin is essential for formation of collagen.)

Cousins was elated. He could sleep without pain. He knew he was going to make it back all the way. After several months of gradual improvement he was able to return to his old job at the *Saturday Review* full time.

REFERENCES

Chapter 1

1. Asimov, Isaac. *Asimov's Biographical Encyclopedia of Science and Technology*, second revised edition. Doubleday & Company, Garden City, NY. 1982. p. 1.
2. Herodotus. *The Histories*. Translated by Aubrey de Selincourt, Penguin Books, Ltd. Baltimore, MD, 1959, p. 132.
3. Wheeler, Talboys. *The Geography of Herodotus*, Longman, Brown, Green, and Longmans, London, 1954.
4. Dubberstein, Waldo H. *Mesopotamia*. The World Book Encyclopedia, Field Enterprises Educational Corporation, Chicago. Vol. 13. p. 345-346; vol. 17, p. 780.
5. Sanford, Eva Mathews. *The Mediterranean World in Ancient Times*. The Ronald Press Company, New York. 1951, p. 45.
6. Kramer, Samuel Noah. *History Begins at Sumer*. Doubleday & Company, Garden City, NY 1959. p. 60-64.
7. World Book Encyclopedia.
8. Roaf, Michael. *Cultural Atlas of Mesopotamia and the Ancient Near East*, Faith on File. New York. 1990.

Chapter 2

1. Lucas. *A Short History of Civilization*
2. Dubos, R. *Man, Medicine, and Environment*. The New America Library, New York. 1969.
3. Roaf, Michael. *Cultural Atlas of Mesopotamia and the Ancient Near East*. Equinox (Oxford) Ltd, Musterlin House, Oxford, England. 1990.

4. Kelly, Emerson Crosby, M.D., Introduction. *The Theory and Practice of Medicine by Hippocrates*. Citadel Press, New York, 1964, by arrangement with The Williams & Wilkins Co., USA.

Chapter 3

1. Asimov, Isaac. *Asimov's Biographical Dictionary of Science and Technology*, 2nd revised ed., Garden City, New York, Doubleday & Company, Inc., 1982.

Chapter 4

1. M. Levey. Medieval Arabic Toxicology. 1966.

Chapter 5

1. Anon. *Peering beyond the light barrier*. Science 314: 1854. Dec. 22, 2006.
2. Anon. *Seeing the Unseeable*. Chemical Heritage, Fall, 2009, p. 19.
3. Maugh II, Tomas H. *James Hillier, 91; designed first practical electron microscope*. Los Angeles Times, January 23, 2007, p. B8.
4. Spence, John C.H. *High Resolution Electron Microscopy*, 3rd ed. Oxford University Press, 2009.
5. Asimov, Isaac. *Asimov's Biographical Dictionary of Science and Technology*, 2nd revised ed., Garden City, NY, Doubleday & Company, Inc. 1982.

Chapter 6

1. Asimov, Isaac. Asimov's Chronology of Science & Discovery (updated and illustrated). Harper Collins, New York. 1994, p. 156.
2. Asimov, p. 156-157.
3. Asimov, p. 157-158.

Chapter 7

1. Asimov, Isaac. Asimov's Biographical Encyclopedia of Science and Technology, second revised edition, Doubleday & Company, Garden City, NY.
2. Asimov, Isaac. Asimov's Biographical Encyclopedia of Science and Technology. Second revised edition, Doubleday & Company, Inc., Garden City, NY. 1982.
3. Asimov, Isaac. Asimov's Chronology of Science & Discovery. Harper Collins Publishers, New York, 1994.
4. Dubos, Rene. Pasteur and Modern Science. Anchor Books, Doubleday & Company, Garden City, N.Y. 1960.

Chapter 8

1. Asimov, Isaac. *Asimov's Biographical Encyclopedia of Science and Technology*. Second revised edition, Doubleday & Company, Inc., Garden City, NY. 1982.

Chapter 9

1. Normile, Dennis. *Rinderpest, Deadly for Cattle, Joins Smallpox as a Vanquished Disease.* Science Vol. 330 p. 435, October 22, 2010.

Chapter 10

1. Dubos, Rene. *Pasteur and Modern Science*, Doubleday & Company, Inc., Garden City, NY. 1960, pp. 121, 122
2. Ibid.
3. Haggard, Howard W., The Doctor in History. Dorset Press, New York. 1989, p. 363.
4. Mainly from a list in Berkow, Robert, et al, *The Merck Manual*, Merck Research Laboratories, Division of Merck & Co., Inc., Whitehouse Station, N.J., 1997, p. 846.

Chapter 11

1. Asimov, Isaac. *Asimov's Biographical Dictionary of Science and Technology*, 2nd revised ed., Garden City, NY, Doubleday & Company, Inc. 1982.

Chapter 13

1. Herms, William B., *Medical Entomology*, 3rd edition. The Macmillan Company, New York. 1939, p. 198.
2. Howard, L. O., An Experiment Against Mosquitoes. Insect Life, vol. 5, No. 1, pp. 12-14, 1892.
3. Salyers, Abigail A. and Dixie D. Whitt. *Revenge of the Microbes*. ASM Press, Herndon, VA, 2005, p. 149.
4. Roberts, Leslie and Martin Enserink. *Did They Really Say…Eradication?* Science: 318, December 7, 2007, p. 1544-1545.
5. Reuters. *Tearful Gates bids farewell to Microsoft*. The Orange County Register, June 28, 2008. News 24.
6. Kilpatrick, Andrew. *Of Permanent Value*. The story of Warren Buffett, revised edition. AKPE Financial Center, North Birmingham, Alabama, 1996.
7. Roberts, Leslie, *New Malaria Plan Called Ambitious by Some, Unrealistic by Others*. Science, Vol. 322, pp 26-27, 3 October, 2008.

Chapter 14

1. Dickerson, James I. *Yellow Fever*. Prometheus Books, Amherst, NY, 2006.

Chapter 15

1. Tortora, Gerard J., Berdell R. Funke, and Christine L. Case. *Microbiology, An Introduction*, 4th ed. p. 570. The Benjamin/Cumings Publishing Company, Inc., Redwood City, CA. 1992.

2. Berkow, Robert, Editor-in-Chief. *The Merck Manual of Medical Information*, pp. 893-894, Merck Research Laboratories, Merck & Co. Inc., Whitehouse Station, NJ, 1997.
3. Asimov Isaac. *Asimov's Biographical Dictionary of Science and Technology*, 2nd revised ed., Garden City, NY, Doubleday & Company, Inc. 1982.
4. Dobson, Mary. *Disease*, pp. 36-43. Quercus, 21 Bloomsbury Square, London, 2007.
5. *World Book Encyclopedia*, vol. 14, pp. 12-17, Field Enterprises Educational Corporation, Chicago.
6. Herms, William B. *Medical Entomology*. The MacMillan Company, NY, 1930.

Chapter 16

1. Sinnigen, William, Ed., Rome. Collier-Macmillan Canada, Ltd., Toronto, Ontario, 1965
2. McNeill, William H., Plagues and Peoples. Anchor Books, Garden Grove, NY, 1976
3. Simond, P.L., La Propagation de la peste. Ann. Inst. Pasteur, vol. Xii, No. 10: 625-687, 1898
4. Verjbitski, D.T., The part played by insects in the epidemiology of plague. Jour. of Hyg., Vol. viii, p. 162
5. Herms, W. B. Medical Entomology, 3rd ed. The MacMillan Company, New York, 1930.
6. Pielou, E. C., After the Ice Age. The return of life to glaciated North America, University of Chicago Press, Chicago, Ill. 1992
7. Ziegler, Philip, The Black Death, Bramley Books, an imprint of Quadrillion Publishing, Ltd., Godalming, Surrey, 1998.
8. Porter, Roy. The Greatest Benefit to Mankind, W. W. Norton, New York, 1997, p. 123
9. Philip Ziegler, The Black Death, pp 31-37
10. Asimov, Isaac. Asimov's Chronology of Science and Discovery. Harper Collins, New York, 1994.
11. Porter, Roy, Ed., The Greatest Benefit to Mankind.

Chapter 17

1. Salyers, Abigail, A., and Dixie D. Whitt. Revenge of the Microbes, ASM Press, Herndon, VA, 2005.
2. Asimov, Isaac. *Asimov's Biographical Dictionary of Science and Technology*, 2nd revised ed., Garden City, NY, Doubleday & Company, Inc. 1982.

Chapter 18

1. Salyers, Abigail A. and Dixie D. Witt. *Revenge of the Microbes*. ASM Press, Herndon, VA, 2005.
2. Anand, Geeta. *A Woman's Drug-Resistant TB Echoes Around the World.* Wall Street Journal September 8-9, 2012, p. A1.
3. Leslie Mitch. *Germs Take a Bite Out of Antibiotics.* Science 320: 33, April 4, 2008.

Chapter 19

1. Dubos, René, *Pasteur and Modern Science* (Garden City, NY: Doubleday & Company, 1960), pp. 23-39.
2. Asimov, Isaac, Asimov's Biographical Encyclopedia of Science and Technology, 2nd revised ed. (Garden City, NY: Doubleday & Company, 1982), pp. 421-425.
3. Stinson, Stephen C., "Chiral Drugs," *Chemical & Engineering News.* October 9, 1995, pp. 44-74; p. 49.
4. Windholz, Martha, ed., The Merck Index, ninth ed. (Rahway, NJ: Merck & Co., Inc, 1976), p. 6346.
5. Stein, Gary S., Janet L. Stein, Andre J. van Wijnen, and Jane B. Lian, "The Maturation of a Cell," *American Scientist* **84** (January-February, 1996), pp. 28-37.
6. Petsko, Gregory A. "On the Other Hand…," *Science* **256** (June 5, 1992), pp. 1403-1404.
7. Jon Cohen, "Getting All Turned Around Over The Origins of Life on Earth," *Science* **267** (March 3, 1995), pp. 1265-1266.

8. Cronin, John R., and Sandra Pizzerello, "Enantiomeric Excesses in Meteoritic Amino Acids," *Science* 275 (February 14, 1997), pp. 951-955.
9. Bradley, David, "A New Twist in the Tale of Nature's Asymmetry," *Science* **264** (May 13, 1994), p. 908.
10. Rawls, Rebecca, "Stereoselective Studies Probe DNA-carcinogen Interactions," *Chemical & Engineering News*, March 10, 1997, pp. 45-48.
11. Stinson, 1995, p. 45.
12. Stinson, Stephen C., "Chiral Drugs," *Chemical & Engineering News*, September 28, 1992, pp. 46-80; p. 47.
13. Stinson, 1992, p. 60.
14. Stinson, 1995, p. 46.

Chapter 20

1. FDA Papers, vol. 1, No. 1, February, 1967
2. Jansen, Wallace F. *America's First Food and Drug Laws*, FDA Consumer, June, 1975, pp. 12-19.
3. Goodman, Lewis S. and Alfred Gilman *The Pharmacological Basis of Therapeutics*, The Macmillan Co., London and Toronto, 1970.
4. Peterson, Jonathon, *AIDS, Industry, Congress, Put FDA on a Fast Track*. Los Angeles Times, November 20, 2004.
5. Hileman, Bette. *FDA Lambasted for Lax Inspections*. Chemical & Engineering News, July 23, 2007, p. 11.
6. Alonso-Zaldivar, Ricardo. *FDA's Fast Track for Medications called "Broken."* Los Angeles Times, June 1, 2005, p. A10.
7. Wolfe, Sidney M. *From the Desk of Sidney M. Wolfe, M.D.*, Public Citizen, Washington, D.C.

Chapter 21

1. Xin Hao and Richard Stone. *Chinese Probe Unmasks High Tech Adulteration with Melamine*. Science 322: 1310-1311. 28 November, 2008.

2. Anon. *Chemical Combo Made Pet Food Deadly*. Chem & Eng News November 19, 2007, p. 43
3. Kraul, Chris. *Panama Agencies prepared 'Medicine' has Deadly Effects*. Los Angeles Times, June 2, 2007, p. A3.
4. Magnier, Mark. *Chinese Applaud Execution of Former Drug Safety Chief*. Los Angeles Times July 11, 2007, p. A1.
5. Ibid.
6. Tremblay, Jean-Francois. *China Executives Stand Trial for Manufacturing Lethal Drug*. Chem. & Eng. News August 20, 2007, p. 11.
7. Ibid.
8. Alonso-Zaldivar, Richard. *FDA Says Chinese Fish Tainted*. Los Angeles Times June 29, 2007, p. C1.
9. Zajac, Andrew. *FDA Sued Over Heparin Seizures*. Los Angeles Times October 20, 2001, p. B4.
10. Rovner, Sophie L. *Silver Lining in Melamine Crisis. Chem & Eng News, May 25, 2009, pp. 36-38.*

Chapter 22

1. Haggard, Howard W. *The Doctor in History*. Dorset Press, New York. 1989. p. 267-268.
2. Atkinson, D. T. *Magic, Myth and Medicine*. Fawcett Publications, Inc., Greenwich, CT, 1956, p. 49.
3. Atkinson, p. 115.
4. Janssen, Wallace F. *America's First Food and Drug Laws*, FDA Consumer, June, 1975, pp. 12-19.
5. Atkinson, p. 153
6. Haggard, *The Doctor in History*, p. 243.
7. Haggard, *From Medicine Man to Doctor*, p. 342-343.
8. Haggard, p. 336.
9. Haggard, p. 292
10. Haggard, *The Doctor in History*, p. 248.

Chapter 23

1. Haggard, Howard W., M.D. *Devils, Drugs and Doctors*. Pocket Books, Inc., New York, NY, pp. 142-144.
2. Hamlin, Christopher. *Deep Doo-Doo*. American Scientist 97: March-April 2009, pp. 156-160.
3. Berkow, Robert, M.D. *The Merck Manual of Medical Information*. Merck Research Laboratory, div. of Merck & Co., Inc., White House, Station, NJ 1997.
4. Asimov, Isaac. *Asimov's Biographical Encyclopedia of Science and Technology*. 2nd ed. rev., Doubleday & Company, Inc., Garden City, NY. 1982.
5. George, Rose. *The Unmentionable World of Human Waste and Why*. Metropolitan Books, 2008.

Also (cited by Christopher Hamlin):

George, Rose. *The Big Necessity*. Metropolitan Books, 2008.

Black, Maggie and Ben Fawsett. *The Last Taboo*. Earthscan, 2008.

Benidickson, Jamie. *The Culture of Flushing*. A Social and Legal History of Sewage. UBC Press, 2007.

Chapter 24

1. Baum, Rudy M. *The Energy Commons, Part 2*, p. 5 Chem & Eng News, November 20, 2006.

Chapter 25

1. Hoffman, Abraham. *Vision or Villainy: Origins of the Owens Valley-Los Angeles Water Controversy*. Texas A&M University Press, 1981. Fictionalized in the movie *Chinatown*.

2. The World Book Encyclopedia, Vol. 9, p. 399. Field Enterprise Educational Corp, Chicago, IL.
3. Walker, Jim. *Pacific Electric Red Cars*. Arcadia Publications, Charleston, SC., 2006.
4. Crump, Spencer. *Ride the Big Red Cars: How Trolleys Helped Build Southern California*. Trans Anglo Books, Los Angeles, CA, 1965.

Chapter 26

1. Pimentel, David and Marcel Pimentel. *Food, Energy, and Society*, revised edition. University of Colorado, 1996, pp 285, 286.
2. Borlaug, Norman. *Feeding a Hungry World*. Science **318**: 359. 19 October 2007.
3. Brown, Lester R. *Outgrowing the Earth*. W.W. Norton & Company, New York and London, 2004.
4. Dowswell, Christopher. *Norman Ernest Borlaug* (1914-2009) Science **326**: 381, 16 October 2009.
5. Stokstad, Erik. The Famine Fighter's Last Battle. Science **324**: 710-712, 8 May 2009.
6. Hovmoller, Mogens, Stovring, Stephanie Waltrer, and Annemarie Fejer Justesen. *Escalating Threat of Wheat Rusts*. Science **329**: 369, 23 July 2010.
7. Hess, Glenn. *Ethanol Wins Big in Energy Policy*. Chemical & Engineering News, September 12, 2005.
8. Kennedy, Donald. *Mixed Grill*, Science **317**: 1145, 31 August, 2007.
9. Bourne Jr., Joel K. *Green Dreams*, Photographs by Robert Clark. National Geographic October 2007: 38-59
10. Dolan, Jack, State funds promised to ethanol firm. Los Angeles Times August 28, 2010, p. AA1.
11. Bourne, Jr., Joel K. *Biofuels: Boon or Boondoggle?* Photographs by Robert Clark. National Geographic October 2007, *Green Dreams*, pp. 38-59.
12. Stork, William. *A Great Time to Make Fertilizers*, Chemical & Engineering News May 14, 2007, p. 30.
13. Murdock, Deroy. *Ethanol Folly Creating Hungrier, Angrier World*, Orange County Register April 18, 2008, p. Local 27.

14. Eligon, John and Matthew L. Wald. *Ethanol's days of promise and prosperity are fading.* Orange County Register, March 17, 2013.
15. White, Ronald D. *U.S. could cut vehicles' fuel use by 80%, study says.* Los Angeles Times, March 20, 2013.
16. Gieger, Kim. *Sugar at Center of Bitter Fight.* Los Angeles Times, August 6, 2012, p. B1.
17. Lopez, Ricardo. *USDA buying meat to aid farmers.* Los Angeles Times, August 14, 2012, p. B2.
18. Peters, Mark. *Prices Surge as Drought Stunts Corn Crop.* The Wall Street Journal, August 11/12, 2012, p. A2.
19. Godfrey, H. Charles J. *Food and Biodiversity.* Science vol. 333, September 2, 2011, pp 1231-1232.
20. Guin, Jeff. *To Feed a World.* Chemical Heritage, Spring 2012, p. 11
21. Ridley, Matt. *The Rational Optimist.*
22. Monsanto Magic.
23. Jakab, Spencer. *More Monsanto Magic Likely to Be Reaped.* Wall Street Journal April 4, 2012, p. C1.
24. Anon. *End Product.* Chemical Heritage Spring 202, p. 48.
25. Asimov, Isaac. *Asimov's Biographical Encyclopedia of Science and Technology*, 2nd revised edition, p. 781.
26. Asimov, p. 610
27. Foster, Steven and Rebecca L. Johnson. *Desk Reference to Nature's Medicine* p. 366-367.

Chapter 27

1. Asimov, Isaac. *Asimov's Biographical Encyclopedia of Science and Technology*, 2nd rev. ed., 1982, Doubleday & Company, Inc., Garden City, NY.
2. Ibid
3. Dully, Howard. *My Lobotomy.*
4. Anon. *Psychiatry, An Industry of Death.* The Citizens Commission on Human Rights, Los Angeles. Undated.
5. Breggin, Peter R., MD. *Toxic Psychiatry*, St. Martin's Press, 1994, p. 53, 262.

6. Breggin, Peter R. *The Anti-depressant Fact Book*, Da Capo Life Long Member of Persius Books, 2001, p. 156.
7. Breggin, *Toxic Psychiatry*, p. 6.
8. Allen, Elena A., et al., *Transcranial Magnetic Stimulation Elicits Coupled Neural and Hemodynamic Consequences*. Science 317: 1918-1921, 28 Sept. 2007.
9. Miller, Greg. *Uncovering Magic in Magnetic Brain Stimulation*. Science 317: 1846, 28 Sept 2007.
10. Quoted by Peter Breggin in *Toxic Psychiatry*, p. 56, referring to Sterling, Peter, *Psychiatry's Drug Addiction*, New Republic, March 3, 1979
11. Goodman, Louis S., and Alfred Gilman, *The Pharmacological Basis of Therapeutics*, 4th ed., 1970, p. 155.
12. Warren, Jennifer, *Mental Ills Rife in Prisons, Jails*. Los Angeles Times, September 7, 2006, p. B3.
13. Levey, Noam N., *Reform Is Locked out of Juvenile Hall*, Los Angeles Times, September 21, 2006, p. A1.
14. Schmidt, Charles. *Putting the Brakes on Psychosis*. Science: 316: 976-977, May 18, 2007

Chapter 28

1. Asimov, Isaac. *Asimov's Biographical Encyclopedia of Science and Technology*, 2nd rev. ed., Doubleday & Company, Inc., Garden City, NY. 1982.

Chapter 29

1. Miles, Steven H., M.D. *Oath Betrayed*. Torture, medical complicity, and the war on terror. Random House, Inc., New York. 2006.
2. Quoted by Harry Bruinius, *Better for All the World*, Alfred A. Knoph, New York, 2006.
3. Williams, Carol I. *Scholars Look at 'Supreme Mistakes'* Los Angeles Times, April 2, 2011, p. AA3.

4. Egra S. Gosney and Paul Popenoe. *Sterilization for Human Betterment: A Summary of Results of 6,000 Operations in California, 1909-1929.* The Macmillan Company, New York, 1931.
5. Bruinius, Harry. *Better for All the World*, Vintage Books, Div. of Random House, New York, 2007, p. 15, 56, 129, 154, 191.
6. Bruinius, p. 17
7. Bruinius, p. 190-191

Chapter 30

1. Harris, Whitney R. *Tyranny on Trial*, revised edition. Southern Methodist University Press, Dallas. 1999.
2. Shah, Sonia, *The Body Hunters.* The New Press, New York, 2006.
3. Katz, Jay. *The Education of the Physician-Investigator*, p. 311, In Paul A. Freund. ed., *Experimentation with Human Subjects*, George Braziller, New York, 1970.
4. Porter, Roy. *The Greatest Benefit to Mankind.* W.W. Norton & Company, New York. 1997.

Chapter 31

1. Amato, Ivan. *Genes take a Backseat.* Chemical & Engineering News, April 6, 2009, p. 28-31.
2. Riddihough, Guy and Laura M. Zahn. *What Is Epigenetics? Science 330: 611, 29 October 2010.*
3. Kaiser, Jocelyn. *Epigenetic Drugs Take On Cancer.* Science 330: 576-578, 29 October 2010.
4. Heijmans BT, Tobi EW, Stein AD, Putter H, Blauw GJ, Sussuer ES, Slagboom PE, Lumey, LH. *Persistent epigenetic differences associated with prenatal exposure to famine in humans.* Proc. Natl. Acad, Sci. USA 2008, Nov 4,105(44): 17046-9
5. Paul, Annie Murphy. *Origins: How the Nine Months Before Birth Shape the Rest of Our Lives.* Free Press, 2010.
6. Remmel, Ethan. *Nurture Before Birth.* American Scientist 99: 160-161. 2010.

7. Agin, Dan. *More Than Genes: What Science Can Tell Us About Toxic Chemistry, Development, and the Risk to Our Children.* Oxford University Press, 2009.

Chapter 32

1. Harris, Sheldon H. *Factories of Death. Japanese Biological Warfare, 1932-1945, and the American Coverup*, Revised Edition. Routledge (Imprint of Taylor & Francis Group), New York, NY, 2002.
2. The World Book Encyclopedia, vo. 20. *World War II, Japan, Pacific,* pp. 392-412. Field Enterprise Educational Corporation, Chicago, 1967.
3. Moore, Kevin. *Forsaken Heroes of the Pacific War. One Man's True Story.* Los Angeles Times, August 17, 2011, p. AAS.
4. The World Book, Vol. 1, *Atomic Bomb*, pp. 828-831.
5. Harris, p xxvi.
6. Harris, p xxviii.
7. Elliot, Helen. *He Has Quite a Story to Tell.* Los Angeles Times January 26, 2007, p. 9
8. Harris, p. 181.
9. Harris, p. 182-298.
10. Harris, p. 278-279
11. Harris, p. 280
12. The World Book, Vol. 7, p. 354.
13. Guttentag, Bill and Dan Sturman. *Revisionism Tokyo-style.* Los Angeles Times, January 18, 2013. (Guttentag and Sturman directed the documentary film "Nanking" which won a Peabody Award in 2009).

Chapter 33

1. Gwin, Peter. *A Mouse for All Seasons.* National Geographic, April. 2008.
2. Wikipedia, The Free Encyclopedia.

3. Prinzmetal, M. On the Human Treatment of Charity Patients, Medical Tribune, September 22, 1965. Quoted by Jay Katz. *The Education of the Physician-Investigator*, p. 311, In Freund, Paul A. *Experimentation with Human Subjects*, George Braziller, New York, 1970.
4. Breggin, Peter R, MD. *The Antidepressant Fact Book*, p. 156. Da Capo Press, Member of the Perseus Books Group, 2001.
5. Shah, Sonia. *The Body Hunters*, pp. 65-67. The New Press, New York, 2006.

Chapter 34

1. Golomb, Beatrice Alexandra. *Acetylcholinesterase inhibitors and the Gulf War illnesses*. PNAS vol. 105, No. 11, March 18, 2008, pp. 4295-4300.
2. Hanson, David, *Panel Validates Gulf War Ills*. Chemical and Engineering News, November 24, 2008, p. 8.
3. Engel, Mary and Thomas H. Maugh II, *Panel says vaccine, pesticides caused Gulf War syndrome*. Los Angeles Times, November 18, 2008, p. A1.
4. *Physicians Desk Reference*, 58th edition, Thompson PDR, Montvale, NJ, 2004.
5. Goodman, Louis S. and Alfred Gilman. *The Pharmacological Basis of Therapeutics*, 4th ed., The MacMillan Company, London, Toronto, 1970.
6. Holmstedt, B., The Ordeal of Old Calabar: The pageant of *Physostigma venenosum* in medicine, in plants in the development of modern medicine. In *Plants in the Development of Modern Medicine*. Swain, T., ed., Harvard University Press, Cambridge, Mass. 1972.
7. Dragstedt, C. A. *Trial by Ordeal*, Quat. Bul. Northwest University Medical School 19: 137-141, 1945.
8. Goodman, Louis S. and Alfred Gilman. *The Pharmacological Basis of Therapeutics*, 4th ed., The MacMillan Company, London, Toronto, 1970, p 442-465.
9. Ball, W.L., et. al., Canadian Jour. Of Biochemistry and Physiology 22: 440. 1954.

10. Neubert, D., and J. Schaefer, Arch. Exptl. Pathol. Pharmakol. 233: 151. 1958.
11. Welch, R. M. and J. M. Coon, Journ Pharmacol. Exptl. Therap.: 144: 192. 1964
12. Barry, W. K. and Davies, D. R., Use of Carbamates and Atropine in the Protection of Animals Against Poisoning by 1,2,2 trimethyl propyl methyl phosphonofluoridate. Biochem. Pharmacol 19: 927, 1970.
13. Dorough, H. W., Effect of Temic on Methylparathion Toxicity to Mice. Texas Agricultural Exp. Sta. Progress Rept. No. 2771: 6. 1970.
14. Kuht, B. J. and H. W. Dorough. Carbamate Insecticides: Chemistry, Biochemistry, and Toxicology. CRC Press, Inc., Cleveland, Ohio. 1976.
15. O'Brian, R. D., *Insecticides, Action and Metabolism.* Academic Press, New York, 1967.
16. Goodsell, David S. *Our Molecular Nature.* Copernicus, imprint of Springer-Verlag, New York, 1996.
17. Cited by Moreno, p. 272, also: Miller, Claire Alda. *Gulf War Guinea Pigs: Is Informed Consent Optional During War?* Journal of Contemporary Health Law and Policy 13: 199-232. 1996.
18. Moreno, Jonathon D. *Undue Risk.* Secret State Experiments on Humans. W. H. Freeman and Company, New York. 1999, 2000, p. 270.

Chapter 35

1. Hilton, James. *Lost Horizon.* William Morrow & Company, Inc. 1933.
2. Wikipedia, the free encyclopedia, 1-30-2011.
3. Brown-Séquard, C. E. *Des effets produits chez l'omme par dez injections souscutane'es d'un liquide retire' des testicules fraise cobaye et de chien,* C. r. Se'anc. Soc. Biol. I: 420-430, 1889.
4. Goodman, Louis D. and Alfred Gilman. *The Pharmacological Basis of Therapeutics.* The Macmillan Company, London, 1970. p. 1571

5. Voronoff, S. *Testicular grafting from ape to man.* Brentano, Ltd, London, 1929.
6. Hamilton, J. B. and G. E. Mestler, *Morality and survival: comparison of eunuchs with intact men and women in a mentally retarded population,* J. Gerontology 24: 395-411. 1969.
7. McCay, C.M., M.F. Crowell, and L. A. Maynard, *The effect of retarded growth upon length of life span and upon ultimate body size.* J. Nutr. 10: 63-79, 1935.
8. Miller, D.S. and P. R. Payne, *Longevity and protein uptake,* Exp. Gerontol. 3: 231-234, 1968.
9. Ross, M. H. and G. Bras, *Dietary preference and diseases of age,* Nature 250: 263-265. 1974.
10. Moment, Gairdner B., *The Ponce de Leon Trail Today,* Bioscience 25, No. 10: 623-628. October 1975.
11. Anon. *Dietary restrictions in Drosophila,* Science 303: 1610-1612, March 12, 2004.
12. Cassiday, Laura A., *The curious case of caloric restriction,* C&EN August 3, 2009, pp. 36-38.
13. Ingram, D.K., et. al. *Dietary restriction and aging. The initiation of a primate study.* J. Gerontol. 45: B148-B163. 1990.
14. J. W. Kemnitz, et. al. *Dietary restriction of adult male monkeys.* Design, methodology, and primary findings from the first year of study. J. Gerontol. 48: B17-B26. 1993.
15. C&EN July 13, 2009, p. 26; Nature 2009, 460, 392; and Science 326: 1602-1603. December 18, 2009.
16. Frey, Bruno S. *Happy People Live Longer.* Science 331: 542-543. February 4, 2011.

Chapter 36

1. Brown, Barbara. *New Mind, New Body.* Harper & Row, New York, 1974, p. 420.
2. Moyer, Bill. *Healing and the Mind,* Doubleday, New York 1995, pp. 7-23. Quotes Thomas Delbanco, *The Healing Roles of Doctor and Patient.*
3. Moyer, pp. 115-143.

4. Benson, Herbert. *Mind/Body Effect*. Simon and Schuster, New York, 1979, pp. 75-76.
5. Hearn, Michael Patrick, Selections and Introduction. Illustrated Works of Mark Twain. Random House, New York, MCMLXXIX.
6. Canon, Walter B. *The Wisdom of the Body* (New York: W. W. Norton, 1963).
7. Cannon, W. B. "Voodoo Death," *American Anthropologist* 44 (1944): 169-81 (cited by Herbert Benson, Timeless Healing, 1996, p. 40)
8. Cannon, W. B., *Bodily Changes in Pain, Hunger, Fear and Rage: An Account of Recent Researches into the Function of Emotional Excitement*, 2nd ed. (New York: D. Appleton and Company, 1929).
9. Benson, Herbert, with Marg Stark, *Timeless Healing: The Power and Biology of Belief* (New York: Simon & Schuster, 1996).
10. The World Book Encyclopedia, Field Enterprise Education Corp., Chicago, IL, 1967, Vol. 17 pp. 53, 54, 259.
11. Brown, pp. 420-421.
12. Chopra, Deepak, *Perfect Health: The Complete Mind/Body Guide* (New York: Random House, 1991).
13. Perry, Tony, "Rich, So Restless," *Los Angeles Times Magazine*, September 7, 1997, pp. 27-30, 51-54.
14. Benson, H., *The Relaxation Response* (New York: William Morrow, 1975).
15. Benson, Herbert, with Marg Stark, *Timeless Healing: The Power and Biology of Belief* (New York: Simon & Schuster, 1996).
16. Benson, H., and M. D. Epstein, "The Placebo Effect—A Neglected Asset in the Care of Patients," *Journal of the American Medical Association* 232 (1975): 1225-1227.
17. Fink, David Harold, *Release From Nervous Tension* (New York: Simon and Schuster, 1943).
18. Alvarez, Walter C. *Live At Peace With Your Nerves* (Englewood Cliffs, NJ: Prentice-Hall.

Chapter 37

1. The World Book Encyclopedia, Field Enterprise Educational Corporation, Chicago, 1936, Vol. 12, p. 436-7.

2. Asimov, Isaac. *Asimov's Guide to the Bible, Two Volumes in One.* Avenal Books, New York, 1981.
3. Channing, George, "What is a Christian Scientist? In Leo Rosten, ed., *A Guide to the Religions of America* (New York: Simon and Schuster, 1955), pp. 21-30; quotes from pp. 22, 23.
4. The World Book, vol. 6, p. 46.
5. Haggard, Howard W. *From Medicine Man to Doctor.* Dover Publications, Inc., Mineola, NY. 2004 Originally published entitled *Devils, Drugs and Doctors: The Story of the Science of Healing from Medicine Man to Doctor.* Harper Brothers, New York and London, 1929.
6. Holmes, Ernest, *The Science of Mind* (New York: Dodd, Mead & Company, 1938), p. 30.
7. Holmes, Ernest, *This Thing Called You* (New York: Dodd, Mead & Company, 1948).
8. Holmes, Ernest Shurtleff, *Creative Mind and Success* (New York: Dodd, Mead & Company, 1943).
9. Peale, Norman Vincent. *The Power of Positive Thinking* (Englewood Cliffs: Prentice-Hall, 1952.
10. Peale, Norman Vincent, *You Can If You Think You Can* (Carmel, NY: Guideposts Associates, Inc., 1974).
11. Fox, Emmet, *The Golden Key* (Marina del Rey, CA: Devores & Co., 1991).
12. Fox, Emmet, *Stake Your Claim* (New York: Harper & Brothers, 1952)
13. Benson, Herbert, M.D. with Marg Stark. *Timeless Healing*, The Power and Biology of Belief. Fireside, New York, 1997, pp. 25-45.
14. Mark 11: 24.
15. Proverbs 3: 5.
16. Neville, Awakened Imagination (Los Angeles: C & J Publishing Company, 1954), p. 20.
17. Benson, Herbert, M.D. with Miriam Z. Klipper. *The Relaxation Response.* Avon Books, New York, 1975.
18. Moyers, Bill, *Healing and the Mind* (New York: Doubleday, 1993), p. 48.
19. Cousins, Norman. *Anatomy of an Illness as Perceived by the Patient.* WW Norton and Company, New York 1979, pp. 155-156.

20. Cannon, Walter B. *"Voodoo Death,"* Psychosomatic Medicine 19:3, 1957. pp. 182-190.
21. Rossi, Ernest Lawrence. *The Psychobiology of Mind-Body Healing.* Norton, NY, 1993.
22. Murray, Jim, "Divine Course for Discipline of Golf," *Los Angeles Times,* July 31, 1997, p. C1.
23. Baxter, Kevin. *Africa's Juju Stays Off the Field.* Los Angeles Times, June 26, 2010, p. A1.
24. The World Book Encyclopedia, Field Enterprise Educational Corporation, Chicago, 1936.
25. The World Book Encyclopedia, Field Enterprise Educational Corporation, Chicago, 1936, Vol. 17, p. 790.

Chapter 38

1. Isaac Asimov, Asimov's Biographical Dictionary of Science and Technology, Second Revised Edition (Garden City, NY: Doubleday & Company, Inc., 1982), pp. 314-315; 493-494.
2. *The World Book Encyclopedia,* Field Enterprise Educational Corp. Chicago, IL, 1967, Vol. 9, pp. 425-478, Vol. 13 p. 345.
3. Asimov, Isaac pp. 494-495.
4. Brown, Barbara, *New Mind, New Body* (New York: Harper & Row, 1974), p. 342.
5. DeBets, Barbara and Gerard Sunnen, *A Primer of Clinical Hypnosis* (Littleton, MA; PSG Publishing Co., 1985), p. 11
6. Brown, Barbara
7. Hull, Clark L. *Hypnosis and Suggestibility: An Experimental Approach.* Appleton Century, New York, 1933. (Cited by Robert A. Baker, *They Call It Hypnosis.* Prometheus Books, Buffalo, N.Y., 1990 p. 17).
8. Coué, Émile, *Self Mastery Through Conscious Autosuggestion* (New York: American Library Service, 1922), cited by Baker, 1990.
9. Coué, Émile, *My Method* (New York: American Library Service, 1923), cited by Baker, 1990.
10. *Encyclopedia Britannica,* 15th edition, p. 674 (Coué)

11. Hull, Clark L. *Hypnosis and Suggestibility: An Experimental Approach.* Appleton Century, New York, 1933. (Cited by Robert A. Baker, *They Call It Hypnosis.* Prometheus Books, Buffalo, N.Y., 1990 p. 17).
12. Caprio, Frank S and Joseph R. Berger. *Helping Yourself To Self-Hypnosis: A Modern Guide to Self-Improvement and Successful Living,* Englewood Cliffs, NJ. 1963, pp. 24, 29.
13. Weil, Andrew, M.D. *Healthy Aging.* A Life-long Guide to Your Physical and Spiritual Well-Being. Alfred A. Knopf, New York, 2005.
14. Moyers, Bill D. *Healing and the Mind.* Doubleday, New York. 1993, pp. 71-83.
15. Baker, Robert A., *They Call It Hypnosis* (Buffalo, NY: Prometheus Books, 1990).

Chapter 39

1. Ganong, William F. *Review of Medical Physiology.* Lange Medical Publications, Los Altos, CA, 1971, p. 29.
2. Goodsell, David S. *Our Molecular Nature.* Springer-Verlag, New York, 1996, p. 159-161.
3. Campbell, Neil A., et. al. *Biology Concepts and Connections.* 4th ed., Benjamin Cummings, San Francisco, CA, 2003.
4. Brown, Barbara B. *New Mind New Body.* Harper & Row, New York, 1974, p. 313.
5. Berger, Hans *Nevenkr* 87: 527 1929; cited by Brown, p. 313.
6. Brown, p. 312-314.
7. Brown, p. 340.
8. Brown, p. 50-60.
9. Brown, p. 126-130.
10. Brown, p. 390-391.

Chapter 40

1. Cousins, Norman. *Anatomy of an Illness as Perceived by the Patient.* Bantam Books, New York. 1981.

2. Cousins, Norman. *The Celebration of Life*. Bantam Books, New York. 1974.
3. Selye, Hans. *The Stress of Life*. McGraw-Hill Book Company, New York. 1956.

ABOUT THE AUTHOR OF *THE HEALERS*

Kenneth Maxwell was raised on a ranch in a remote area of southern California where he attended a one-teacher grade school. After high school in Riverside, California, and two years at junior college (community college), he attended UC Berkeley and obtained a Bachelor of Science degree with a major in entomology.

While at Berkeley, his advisor, a chemist, encouraged him in his interest in toxicology of pesticides. It led to an award of a graduate scholarship at Cornell University where he received a PhD degree with a joint major in entomology and plant pathology. Following a stint on the faculty at UC agricultural experiment station in Riverside, he moved to a career in the chemical industry where he worked on a variety of projects in research and management for several companies. He returned to academia by joining the faculty of California State University, Long Beach, where he initiated three new courses and directed research projects sponsored by the National Institutes of Health (NIH) and the U.S. Fish and Wildlife Service. He served as chairman of the Research Committee, and chairman of the Radiation Safety Committee. He is now Professor Emeritus at CSULB.

Courses initiated and taught at CSULB:

- Economic Entomology
- Toxicology of Pesticides
- Environmental Toxicology

Books by Kenneth Maxwell:

Chemicals and Life. Dickenson Publ. Co. 1970 (Edited and coauthored)

Environment of Life. Dickenson Publ. Co. 1973, 1976. Brooks-Cole 1980. 1985. (Fourth edition, 1985, coauthored by Dr. Greayer Mansfield-Jones and Dr. Dorothy Mansfield-Jones).

Remember the Armada. A history and genealogy of James B. and Myrtle N. Maxwell. Shumway Family History Service. 1990.

A History and Genealogy of the Family of Kenneth E. and Rosemarie A. Greenwood Maxwell. Shumway Family History Service. 1992.

The Sex Imperative. An Evolutionary Tale of Sexual Survival. Plenum Publishing Corporation. 1994.

A Sexual Odyssey. From Forbidden Fruit to Cybersex. Plenum Publishing Corporation. 1996.

Environmental Toxicology Syllabus. Self-published. Copyright 1976.

www.ingramcontent.com/pod-product-compliance
Lightning Source LLC
Chambersburg PA
CBHW051800170526
45167CB00005B/1821